Magneto Therapy
The Miraculous Healing Power

Rajendar Menen

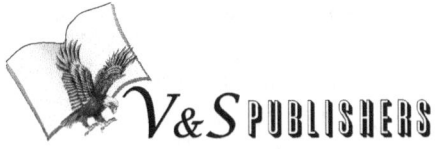

Published by:

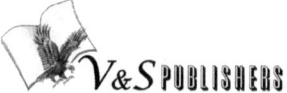

F-2/16, Ansari road, Daryaganj, New Delhi-110002
☎ 23240026, 23240027 • *Fax:* 011-23240028
Email: info@vspublishers.com • *Website:* www.vspublishers.com

Branch: Hyderabad
5-1-707/1, Brij Bhawan (Beside Central Bank of India Lane)
Bank Street, Koti Hyderabad - 500 095
☎ 040-24737290
E-mail: vspublishershyd@gmail.com

Distributors:

▶ **Pustak Mahal®**, Delhi
J-3/16, Daryaganj, New Delhi-110002
☎ 23276539, 23272783, 23272784 • *Fax:* 011-23260518
E-mail: sales@pustakmahal.com • *Website:* www.pustakmahal.com
Bengaluru: ☎ 080-22234025 • *Telefax:* 080-22240209
Patna: ☎ 0612-3294193 • *Telefax:* 0612-2302719

▶ **PM Publications**
- 10-B, Netaji Subhash Marg, Daryaganj, New Delhi-110002
  ☎ 23268292, 23268293, 23279900 • *Fax:* 011-23280567
  E-mail: pmpublications@gmail.com
- 6686, Khari Baoli, Delhi-110006
  ☎ 23944314, 23911979

▶ **Unicorn Books**
Mumbai:
23-25, Zaoba Wadi (Opp. VIP Showroom), Thakurdwar, Mumbai-400002
☎ 022-22010941 • *Telefax:* 022-22053387

© **Copyright:** V&S PUBLISHERS
ISBN 978-93-813848-1-7
Edition: 2011

The Copyright of this book, as well as all matter contained herein (including illustrations) rests with the Publishers. No person shall copy the name of the book, its title design, matter and illustrations in any form and in any language, totally or partially or in any distorted form. Anybody doing so shall face legal action and will be responsible for damages.

Printed at : Parma Offsetters, Okhla, New Delhi

DEDICATION

For Motabhoy Contractor,

who sheltered me from the

sun and the rain and allowed

the words to flow

unencumbered.

Acknowledgements

I wish to thank all the earlier chroniclers of magneto-therapy for their pioneering efforts. It is a difficult subject and yet they managed to get their point across. A big hurrah to Burl Payne, Dr Bansal and all the others who have managed to put magneto-therapy in the upper echelons of alternative healing.

Contents

Preface 7

SECTION I

1. How Magnets are a Healing Tool 11
2. History of Magnets 19
3. The Force of Magnetism 22
4. Types of Magnets 25
5. The Applications 28
6. Some Do's and Don'ts in Diagnosis and Treatment 32
7. Treatments for Specific Ailments 35
8. Some More Research and Treatments 53
9. Duration of Treatment 58
10. How Safe are the Treatments? 60
11. Choice of Magnets 62
12. Magnetisation of Water 68
13. The Spin Force 71
14. Cancer Cure and More Research 73
15. The Beginning of Modern Research 77
16. Electromagnetic Fields 79

17. Magnetic Fields and Living Bodies 84
18. Magnetic Field Surplus Syndrome 87
19. Magneto-Therapy in India 88
20. Curing Complex Ailments with Magneto-Therapy 91

Section II

1. Observations, Treatments and Discoveries 97
2. More Health-Care Attention 99
3. Significance of Biomagnetism 102
4. A Small Trial Raises Hope 103
5. How Does Magneto-Therapy Work? 107
6. Magneto-Therapy and Brain Injury 109
7. Magnets, Minerals and the Human Body 111
8. Hope for Epileptics? 115
9. Therapy of the Future 118

Preface

Magnets are known to all of us. We have played with magnets or used them at some time or the other in our lives. We may have, unwittingly, even come close to magnets at the doctor's office, in some medical examination or the other, and yet not given it a second thought.

Did we ever imagine, even for a microsecond, that magnets are all around us and the very essence of our being? The earth has a magnetic force, the planets have a magnetic force, every little atom in our bodies has a magnetic force all its own. For that matter, every living creature in the solar system has a magnetic force. Its presence is so universal, and so invisible, just like the air we breathe, that it is easily taken for granted.

Let me illustrate this with a simple example. The other day, while researching the book, I was sitting with a friend of mine at a bar. The friend, a well-travelled sports correspondent, is one who goes purely by empirical evidence. He is an agnostic and a complete believer in science. So I broached the subject gently, lest a reprimand sully an otherwise perfect evening.

I told him that I was working on a book on magnets and I had stumbled on an ancient truth that their invisible presence permeated every aspect of our lives. He looked at me with large, disbelieving eyes and suddenly, without a word, bent forward and, with his right hand, pulled out something from his back. It was a tiny magnet strapped to a piece of plaster. "I got this at Heathrow airport," he told me, "and I use it for back and muscular pains. It is very effective."

I was taken aback. My friend continued with some eloquence on the use of magneto-therapy in sport and how he had seen it work on himself with enormously gratifying results. I was, at that time, under the impression that I was researching a secret therapy! But later, as I asked around, I was surprised by the general affirmation given to magneto-therapy.

As I went along and met practitioners, I realised that magneto-therapy had entered the Indian consciousness. Magneto-therapy products were on sale at select outlets and there was a substantial demand for them. Belts, bands, necklaces, earrings and other accessories with magnets worked into them were also commonly used.

This gave me great joy. I realised that I was fortunate to be chosen to document an ancient therapy that was finally being accorded a place by modern science. If, at the end of the book, you will have gleaned something about the use of magnets for better health, the effort will not have been in vain.

—Rajendar Menen

SECTION I
All About Magnets & Magnetism

1. How Magnets are a Healing Tool

As children, we have all been fascinated by pieces of iron that attracted and repelled each other with unimaginable force. We played with the little pieces in awe of the 'magic' they seemed to exude until parents and teachers explained to us that they were 'magnets' and that Nature had invested in them properties to attract and repel.

The entire cosmos, comprising universes and infinite galaxies of stars and planets, is delicately balanced by magnetism. Since man also shares the subtle and crude forces of the cosmos, it makes sense to believe that he must also be balanced by the same magnetism.

Magneto-therapy is a clinical system in which human ailments are treated and cured through the application of magnets to the body. It is a simple, cheap and entirely painless system of treatment with almost no side or after effects. The only tool in the entire treatment process is the magnet.

The earliest mention of the magnet as a healing agent occurs in the Atharvaveda – one of the four Vedas, which contains the treatise on medicine and the art of healing.

It is believed that the builders of pyramids in Egypt were well acquainted with the properties of the magnetic forces and utilised them in the preservation of dead. Queen Cleopatra of Egypt (69-30 BC) is said to have worn a small magnet on her forehead to preserve her beauty. There are innumerable other examples of the use of magnets in ancient times.

The mention of the mineral magnetite appears in Greek writings as early as 80 BC. According to Encyclopaedia Britannica, the Chinese were familiar with the qualities of the magnet as early as the 2nd century. But it was only in the year 1300 AD that the Chinese developed a compass from the magnet. In Europe the first mention of the magnet occurs in a work entitled De Magneta (1600 AD) by William Gilbert. He established that a piece of magnetised iron loses its properties when heated, but regains them on cooling. The compass was invented in Europe much later.

Michael Faraday, the discoverer of electricity, was the first in Europe to study the force of the magnet and he called the area of its influence the magnetic field.

The discovery of the magnet was quite accidental. And if its healing properties were used by the ancients, it was done unwittingly. They were unaware of the magnetic forces in nature and anything awe-inspiring was ascribed to supernatural intervention.

Magneto-therapy was never made an object of scientific investigation till the beginning of the 16th century when a Swiss alchemist and physician P.A. Paracelsus undertook a study and brought to light the healing powers of the magnet. He made the revolutionary observation that the magnet could cure all inflammations, influxes, ulcerations and many diseases of the bowels and uterus. He opined, after considerable investigation, that magnets could be useful both in internal as well as external ailments.

Father Hall, an Austrian Professor of Astronomy in the 18th century, took the cue from Paracelsus and treated nervous men and women by applying magnets to their bodies as remedial tools. Magnetic treatment given by Hall was closely watched by Dr Friedrich Anton Mesmer (1733-1815) of Mesmerism fame. Dr Samuel Hahnemann (1755-1843), the Father of Homeopathy, picked up the baton from there and used the principles of magneto-therapy in the preparation of homeopathic medicines.

All this fuelled enormous research. Magneto-therapy had now come to stay and gained a foothold in the medical interventions of that time.

Dr William Gilbert (1540-1600) of England, the court physician to Queen Elizabeth I, pioneered the scientific study of electricity and magnetism. He was the first to declare that the earth itself was a huge magnet. Michael Faraday (1791-1867) laid the foundations of Biomagnetics and Magneto-chemistry and established that all matter is magnetic in one way or the other and is either attracted or repelled by a magnetic field. In 1862, Louis Pasteur discovered that the earth's magnetic field exercised a positive effect on the growth of plants.

All these discoveries had taken the lid off a hornet's nest. Now there was no stopping the furious pace of further research.

From here, the biomagnetists in America, Russia, Japan, England and France carried out extensive research on the nature and scope of the magnetic field and its effect on living organisms. Thousands of experiments on bacteria, flies, mice, birds, fish, pigeons and rabbits, as well as on plants and tissue cultures, were conducted with amazing results.

It has now been proved that magnets can cure a number of common and serious human ailments without any medicinal aids. Experimenting biomagnetists and practising magneto-therapists have demonstrated that magnetic treatment drives out all types of bodily pains, helps in speedy healing of wounds and fractured bones, dissolves any clots in the blood vessels, washes out stones in kidneys and the gall-bladder and cures diseases like arthritis, asthma, eczema, inflammation, paralysis, polio, slipped disc, spondylitis, stiffness, swelling, tumours etc. There are reports of even cancer being successfully treated in the initial stages with the application of magnets.

Magnets, as we will soon see, have become a convenient, safe, dependable and complementary tool in the treatment of disease.

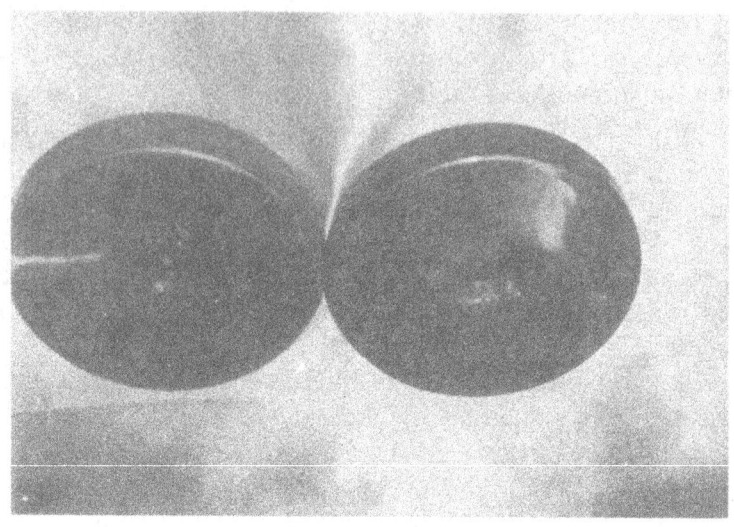

High-power magnets – used to heal many ailments.

Magnets regulate the natural systems of the body and so help the efficacy of any medication being taken. Therefore, while undergoing magneto-therapy, there is no need to discontinue the current mode of treatment.

Magneto-therapy is rooted in natural laws. It is also cheap and easy to use. No lengthy preparations or big money is needed to start and continue with it. A pair of prescribed magnets are the only prerequisites. With it a number of people can be treated for years. Water or any other liquid can be regularly magnetised by the same magnets and used as an accessory to the main line of treatment. If, after years of continuous use, the pair or pairs of magnets lose part of their power, they can be recharged and a renewed span of life given to them. No recurring expenses occur.

Magnets are great time-savers too. Tortuous queues at hospitals are avoided and common ailments can be cured at home.

The application of magnets for about ten minutes daily, in addition to drinking magnetised water everyday, also serves as a preventive against disease and exhaustion.

There is no danger of habit formation with the continued use of magnets. Neither does the magnet lose its effect on the human body after protracted application. There are no side effects either. Even if a high-power magnet has been applied for a time longer than prescribed, the only possible reaction could be slight tiredness immediately after application, and even that is temporary.

An accident started a scientific probe into the effects of magnetism on water. The scientific probes, quite naturally, spilled over to blood too. A few decades ago, Russian technicians and scientists were searching for an easy method to rid the inner walls of pipes of salt deposits. During experiments, they found to their amazement that if magnetised water was passed through the pipes, the hard deposits fell off and were dissolved in water. What's more, further concentration of deposits was restricted and often arrested. The same results were achieved in the radiators of automobiles.

This proved that magnetism somehow transformed simple water into a charismatic liquid. Research also showed that consequent upon the exposure of water to the magnetic field, its temperature, density, surface tension, viscosity and electrical conductivity were affected. Magnetism increased the speed of sedimentation of suspended tiny particles in water and enhanced its conductivity. It hastened the process of ionisation in water.

The study of the effect of magnetism on water naturally attracted the attention of bio-magnetists. Now they took up blood, the most important fluid in the body, for a similar study. The results, again, were amazing.

They found that the magnetic contact immediately activated the iron content in the blood and a weak current was generated. An increase, directly proportionate to the strength of the magnetic field, in the number of centres of crystallisation, was achieved. The process of ionisation (dissociation of atoms or molecules into electrically charged particles) was also hastened.

This freed the blood from the danger of clotting and stimulated easier and more spontaneous flow through the arteries and veins. The magnetic flux created in the blood resulted in an increase in the number of red corpuscles and strengthened the inactive and decayed ones. The movement of haemoglobin in blood vessels was accelerated and calcium and cholesterol deposits in the blood were brought to a minimum.

What was more, it was discovered that magnetism exercised a similar effect on all other fluids in the body. It also helped the secretion of hormones, built new cells and rejuvenated the tissues and exercised a stabilising effect on the genetic code.

Magnetic phenomena have held a strange fascination for the human mind throughout the ages. Lodestone, as the natural deposits of magnetic iron ore were called in ancient times, was the first magnetic material known to man.

The word 'lodestone' or 'loadstone' is derived from the old English word 'load' meaning 'way' because, during the Middle Ages, it was discovered that when a piece of lodestone was suspended by a thread, one end always pointed North and the other South. It was known as the 'Chariot of the South' to the Chinese almost four thousand years ago, and helped them in direction finding.

In ancient Greece and Rome it was known that a piece of loadstone (today called 'magnetite') attracted bits of iron. It was believed that charms made of these stones could attract one's lover; that if the wife of an unfaithful husband were to place a piece of magnetite beneath his pillow, he would have terrible nightmares; that if a piece of magnetite was placed on the head, one could hear the voices of Gods! It was also used as an amulet for headaches, cramps, gout, and a host of other ailments.

In ancient Greece, as legend would have it, while tending his sheep on Mount Ida, a shepherd boy by the name of

Magnes happened to place his iron staff on a piece of rock and found that he couldn't pull it free. 'Magnet' could well have come from Magnes. However, the explanation that is closer to the truth is that the word 'magnet' is derived from Magnesia, a city in Asia Minor (Turkey) where magnetic iron ore was found in abundance.

It is difficult to guess how the ancients understood magnetism of the earth and other celestial bodies in the cosmos and its effect on life and disease. The age-old concept of fasting on new moon and full moon days, when the lunar effect on the liquids and all other fluids is tremendous, has now been scientifically understood. On those days, all the martial humours (the fluid and semi-fluid substances in the body containing iron) are attracted under the influence of the moon and can lead to severe mental and emotional problems. The fasting recommended ensures reduction in body fluids as a precaution against these abnormal effects.

Similarly, our ancestors believed that a person in the last moments of his life should be made to sleep with his head facing the north and feet facing the south to induce magnetic parallelism between the earth and the body. This brought peace, tranquillity, mitigation of pain and less suffering while departing the body.

Some scientists who have been working on the effects of the earth's magnetism as well as the effects of solar flares and sunspot activities have found that these cause disturbances in the earth's magnetism leading to severe biological changes in living beings.

It has also been found that different organs of the human body produce fluctuating magnetic fields due to the different chemical activities in the body. This only proves that every cell in the human body has a specific magnetic value. The highest magnetic field is produced by the brain during sleep followed by the magnetic field of the heart, which can now be precisely measured by science.

It has also been found that the North Pole has antibiotic properties (it can retard or control infection) and the South Pole has energy-giving properties (it can provide warmth and energy to different organs). Therefore, the North Pole has been found useful in diseases where infection is the root cause, while the South Pole has been found more useful in pains, swellings, stiffness, and related problems.

For many years now, artificial magnets made by man have replaced the natural loadstone. Magnets these days have different shapes and different potencies. Some are bar-shaped, horseshoe-shaped, needle-shaped and disc-shaped.

Magneto-therapy, ironically, is both one of the oldest forms of medical treatment and one of the newest! It is only now that this remarkable healing modality is being explored. And it is returning the favour with impressive results.

2. History of Magnets

Magnets have been used in healing for thousands of years. Egyptian nobility were reported to have worn magnetic jewellery to preserve youth and beauty. African tribes used magnetic ores in food preparation. According to Minda Hsu and Chikuo Fong, two modern researchers of biomagnetism, magnetic therapy has been used in China for more than two thousand years. The oldest known medical book, the Chinese Yellow Emperor's Book of Internal Medicine, thought to have been written about 2000 BC, mentions the use of magnets on acupuncture points.

Moving away from the Orient, Aristotle wrote in 300 BC about the use of magnets for healing. Pliny the Younger, a Greek physician, wrote about how diseases were treated in Greece in 100 AD. Galen, a third century Roman physician, observed that magnets were used to rid people of constipation.

In 400 AD, French physicians wrote about the use of magnetic necklaces. The use of magnets continued unabated. In 1530, the physician Paracelsus mentioned using the different poles of a magnet to heal.

More recently, in 1977, the French Royal Society of Medicine appointed two experts to verify the value of magnets in the treatment of disease. After careful scrutiny, the experts were convinced that magnets could really heal.

Slowly, scientific methods and rational thought started gaining ground. Even the cynics realised that magnets, when used properly, are an ideal healing apparatus.

In 1936, Albert Davis rediscovered that the two poles of a magnet have different biological effects. He carried out innumerable experiments on animals, seeds and plants. Davis' basic finding was that one pole stimulated living organisms and the other pole calmed them. In 1948, physicians in the then Soviet Union reported that magnetic treatments could reduce pain after the amputation of limbs. In the 1960s, the Canadian Ministry of Agriculture reported improved germination after grain was exposed to magnetic forces.

The Japanese weren't to be left behind. They began serious medical research and embarked on the large-scale manufacture of magnetic devices including necklaces, bracelets and beads. It is estimated that ten per cent of the Japanese population use magnetic devices for better health. The Japanese Health Ministry has also fully approved magnetic healing, which is a huge industry in Japan.

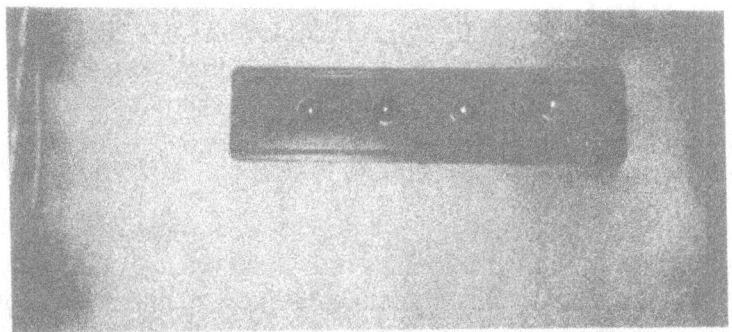

Magnetic ear tops to stimulate the ear, nose and right brain.

Magnetic treatment has now spread to different parts of the world. In Europe, since the 1970s, electrically generated pulsed magnets have been in vogue in health spas. In the US, where conventional medicine has a stranglehold, mainstream medical doctors are routinely using the healing power of magnets in their treatments as an accessory to allopathic medication.

The Swiss physician Marcus Weber, in 1992, describes a study of the results of pulsed magnetic fields on over a thousand patients with acute and chronic problems ranging from inflammation to circulation disorders. Physicians who evaluated the results were amazed by the healing properties of magnets. No side effects were observed either.

3. The Force of Magnetism

Magnetism is universal. It is everywhere. We live and breathe it. It is one of the basic principles of existence. The earth is a huge magnet and its magnetic field can be detected over 100,000 kms away. It is not only the earth but even the human body and the tiniest atoms in nature that are magnets. The sun, moon and other celestial bodies are also giant magnets. So the force of magnetism is all around and within us.

The sun has a magnetic field 100 times greater than that of the earth. The sun's influence on our lives is immeasurable – it cannot be overemphasised. Just like the sun, the moon is also closely linked to our lives. Our calendars are filled with references to the sun and the moon, and science and history are replete with examples of how they affect our lives on an everyday basis. Even the stars are huge magnets and impact our lives and our destinies in strange ways. That's how astrology, the study of the effect of stars and planets on our lives, has taken such a stranglehold on society.

Man is a tiny replica of the cosmos. The human structure and the structure of every living thing, however small and insignificant, is also sustained by the same magnetic force which keeps the cosmos together. People have magnetic fields and can attract and repel others strongly without knowing why. It is not uncommon to hear about somebody having a "magnetic personality" or of some people instantly attracting or repelling one another. This can be attributed to the seemingly invisible magnetic force within and around us. Man's inner nature, the state of his spiritual, mental and emotional health is represented in his magnetic field body. Even the reading of auras and halos are related to the existence of the individual's magnetic field.

The human body is also run by electric impulses, which are generated within the body. During this process, magnetism is simultaneously produced. Every living being possesses some elements of electricity and some properties of associated magnetism. Simply put, electricity and magnetism are the twin manifestations of the same basic energy.

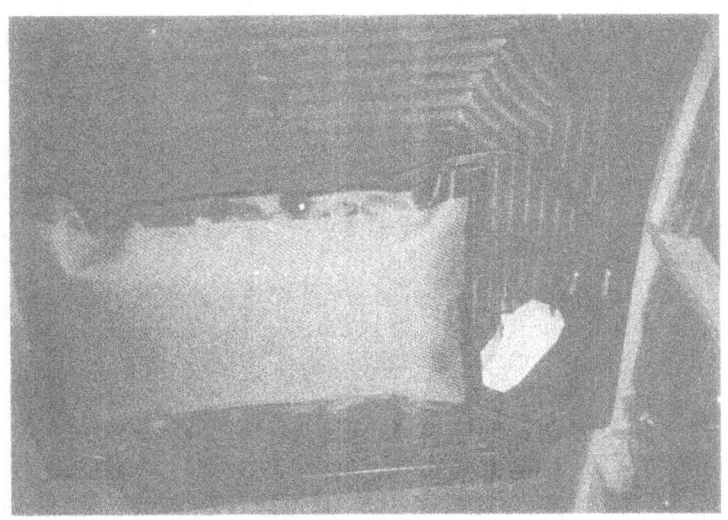

Electro-magnetic body warmer – treats body pain through heat fermentation.

All parts of the body generate electricity for their work. The human body can be compared to an electrical battery and is capable of generating electromagnetic waves at the rate of 80 million cycles per second. Just like electricity, all the organs in the body create their own magnetic fields of varying intensity. The brain creates the strongest electricity and magnetic fields. The magnetic fields fluctuate within the body and mind of the person and are immediately reflected in the magnetic field of the whole body. Now science is able to measure the magnetic fields of individual organs, which is a great help in the diagnosis of different ailments.

The essence is to preserve the balance of the magnetic fields within the body. When they get disrupted for whatever reason, the human body enters a state of dis-ease. Magneto-therapy, in its current sophisticated incarnation, simply attempts to preserve the balance of the magnetic fields within the body with man-made permanent magnets.

4. Types of Magnets

There are many types of magnets. Let's look at them in some detail.

Natural magnets or loadstones are formed when molten lava containing iron or iron oxides cools and is magnetised by the earth's magnetic force. When the lava is molten, it does not exhibit magnetic properties. But when it cools, the tiny molten particles of iron twist around to align with the earth's magnetic poles and are trapped in this position when the iron solidifies.

It is not clear how the earth became a magnet but it is believed that the earth's magnetic force is mostly generated by spinning molten iron within a planet that is also spinning. The magnetic stone found in nature is primarily composed of iron and oxygen. They are found in abundance. Artificial magnets though had to be made by man as science needed magnets in different shapes and varying strengths for a variety of purposes from healing to serious experimentation.

Magnets remained one of nature's mysteries for thousands of years. The only magnets available for a long time were the natural magnets and they were used as compasses. Then, in the 19th century, batteries were developed and a connection between electric current flow and magnetism was discovered. One discovery led to another.

Finally, it was conclusively proved that two wires conducting current and placed side by side will attract each other if the current is in the same direction, or repel if the currents are in the opposite direction.

It was also found that by shaping wire into a coil, the magnetic force around each wire segment would add up to produce a concentrated magnetic force in the centre. These coils were called electromagnets. It was then discovered that the magnetic force in the centre of a coil could be increased by placing a piece of iron inside the coil. Once placed inside a coil, a piece of iron would still hold its magnetic force for a while after the current in the coil was turned off. This was a great discovery. It meant that magnets could now be artificially made. This discovery changed the course of scientific investigation. It leapfrogged generations and new vistas suddenly opened in the world of magnetic applications.

The discovery of electromagnets led to permanent magnets. Magnets are alloys made by adding different metals to finely ground iron, heating the mixture to melting point and then pouring it into moulds of different shapes. Magnets are given an initial magnetisation while still in the molten form but after they are cooled and hardened, they are demagnetised. Prior to being sold at various distribution points, they are remagnetised at room temperature.

Manufactured magnets are much stronger than loadstones. All artificial magnets use iron as the primary ingredient. Iron has 26 electrons. Within the iron atom are a few electrons that are free to change their spin orientation. When external magnetic forces are applied, these new electrons in each atom will align with the applied magnetic force. The aligned magnetic spin fields of adjacent atoms reinforce each other. When enough electrons in enough atoms are organised in this manner, the iron or iron alloy manifests the property we call magnetism.

Magnets can be made in three ways.

One method is by repeated rubbing on a material which can absorb the magnet's power. The other method is the one we just mentioned – the electrical method. But there is a third method too and that is with an instrument called the Magnetiser, which can charge the magnetic material instantly without the use of any wires. It is in vogue in many parts of the world.

Artificial magnets are of two types: permanent magnets and electro-magnets. Permanent magnets remain magnetised permanently once they have been fully charged with electric current. Electro-magnets work only when they are connected with electricity.

All magnets, regardless of size, have two poles – the North Pole and the South Pole. If a large magnet is cut into pieces, each piece will become an independent magnet with poles at either end. The poles are actually the concentrations of magnetism at the two ends of a magnet. Magnetic power is at the highest at the two poles and lowest at the point equidistant from the poles.

Opposite poles attract each other and like poles repel. This proves that the two poles differ in nature and in therapeutic effect too. Magneto-therapy is based on the properties of these two poles.

These poles, it has been discovered, also have different biological effects.

For healing, though, the strength of the magnet is less important than choosing the correct polarity. But how do we measure the strength of magnets?

A magnet exerts a twisting and pulling force on some of the electrons in iron atoms. Since the electrons are bound in atoms, they aren't free to jump out. So the entire piece of iron moves towards the magnet. The force of attraction is called a gauss after the German mathematician Karl Fredrick Gauss. So gauss strength is actually the pulling force measured at the surface of the magnet.

5. The Applications

As we have just mentioned, magnets have two poles – north and south. Now let us see if both the poles, when applied to the body, exercise the same effect. Dr Hahnemann, the founder of Homeopathy, understood this difference and prepared two separate medicines from the two poles for completely different symptoms. Concurrently, scientists also found out that the magnetisation of water with the North Pole neutralised bacteria in it, while the South Pole did just the opposite – it hastened the development of bacteria.

In the early years of magneto-therapy, it wasn't understood why a particular pole proved ineffective in a particular disease while its opposite pole served the purpose. Then sustained research established the fact that the North Pole was effective in diseases caused by bacterial infections, while the South Pole works well in alleviating different kinds of pain.

There were two theories regarding the application of magnetic poles to the body. The unipolar theory advocates the use of a single pole at one time and the bipolar theory believes that the application of both the poles at the same time in the same disease is more effective. The bipolar theory has gained currency and is now being widely practised.

In the application of magnets, there is local treatment and general treatment. In local treatment, the selected pole is applied directly to the affected part of the body.

When the illness is not localised or is extensive, general treatment becomes necessary. In this case, both the poles are brought in touch with the palms of the hands or the soles of the feet. Through the palms and the soles, which are a reservoir of nerve endings, magnetism is instantly carried to every part of the body.

If the illness is in the upper half of the body, the magnets are to be placed under the palms. If the lower half of the body is diseased, then the magnets should be applied to the soles. The frequency of the use of magnets and the cumulative time for which they are used will depend on the gravity of the illness.

The body is a magnet and so has magnetic sides. In treatment, the North Pole has to be applied to the right side and the South Pole to the left side. Similarly, the North Pole should be applied to the upper side and South Pole to the lower side of the body. In the same way, the North Pole should be placed on the front of the body and the South Pole on the back of the body.

But no rule is rigid and it depends on the physician's discretion and the patient's sense of well-being. Magneto-therapists adopt different methods and all cures finally depend on the illness, its severity, the patient and a number of other variables and constants, which we will discuss in the forthcoming chapters.

Magneto-therapy has also adopted the standard leads of electro-cardiography. Positive and negative currents of electricity correspond to the North and South Poles of a magnet. In electro-cardiography both the forearms and the left leg are used. Two tracings are drawn at the same time. Two electrodes, one positive and the other negative, are used. So, from the two forearms and the left leg, three combinations are made: right arm-left arm, right arm-left leg, left arm-left leg. These three combinations are called the standard leads in ECG. Magneto-therapy has adopted this standard leads theory and added two more combinations – the right hand-right foot and the right foot-left foot. Thus, as per the standard leads theory, five methods of the application of magnets are in practice in magneto-therapy.

When magnets have to be applied to several parts of the body, the treatment should start from the upper parts and proceed towards the lower parts. The magnets should first be applied under the palms, then on the back and on the knees and, in the end, under the soles. When high or medium-powered magnets are applied to the palms, the patient should sit on something like a bench or stool and both the magnets should be placed on both sides of the patient or in front of him. The North Pole magnet should be on the right side and the South Pole magnet on the left side. The right palm should be on the North Pole and the left palm on the South Pole.

In another method of application, the North Pole magnet should be kept on the bench or stool and the right palm placed over it. The South Pole magnet can be kept on a wooden plank placed on the ground with the left foot on the South Pole.

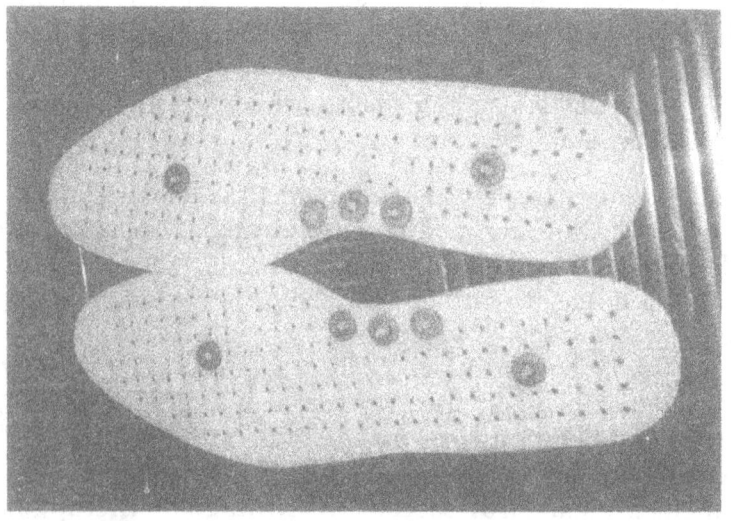

Shoe sole – meant to alleviate rheumatic pains.

In the third method, the palm should be kept on the North Pole magnet placed on the left or right side of the patient. And the sole should be placed on the South Pole magnet placed on the wooden plank on the same side.

With ceramic magnets, the North Pole should be applied to the right side of the body with the patient in a sitting or lying posture. Likewise, the South Pole should be on the left side. It is best to place the feet on a wooden plank.

6. Some Do's and Don'ts in Diagnosis and Treatment

It is apparently quite easy to stimulate healing by applying magnets to the body. But, before that, let us look at some basic principles.

- The South Pole stimulates and promotes healing, growth and activity.

- The North Pole calms, sedates and reduces inflammation.

- Don't treat tumours, cancers or infections with the South Pole at the site of the problem. Since the South Pole stimulates growth, it could stimulate the growth of cancer cells, bacteria or viruses.

- Pregnant women shouldn't be treated around the uterus.

- Those with pacemakers shouldn't be treated with magnets around the chest area.

- Don't use strong magnets around the head, neck, glands or organs for long periods of time everyday.

- Don't treat a condition with magnetism if it worsens when either polarity is applied.

Remember, you can treat any condition with magnets. There are rarely any harmful side effects. But magnetic therapy doesn't seem to help bacterial infections once they have established their presence in the human body.

All biomagnetic aids should be kept away from fire. The patient should preferably avoid anything cold for an hour after the use of belly and knee belts. They shouldn't bathe either for an hour after their use.

The best time for magnetic treatment is in the morning. Early risers can bathe before the treatment and have breakfast after it. It is best to avoid cold food and drink for an hour after applying high-powered magnets. Hot food and drink is allowed. High-powered magnets should not be used immediately after a full meal. Unless watches are magnet-proof, they should not be allowed to come in contact with magnets. If a magnet or pole has been incorrectly selected or applied for an undue length of time, any adverse effect can be neutralised by laying both palms or both feet on a zinc plate.

As we have mentioned earlier and will continue to emphasise in the pages to follow, the duration of treatment differs from person to person and the severity of the ailment. But, generally, some improvement is noticed in a few weeks. If there is no relief at all, then a second opinion should be taken.

Research has proved beyond doubt that the human body is made up of tiny cells, which are tiny magnets in themselves. For good physical health, the equilibrium in the individual magnetic fields and a balance in the magnetic fields of different organs has to be maintained. Any disturbance or abnormal fluctuation in the magnetic field of a particular organ or organs will result in an ailment. A single organ disrupted could well result in the disruption of the whole body.

Normally, all the other systems of medicine introduce chemicals in the form of medication. Magneto-therapy works at the problem by the external application of magnets to the body supplemented by doses of magnetised water. Magneto-therapy activates the liquids in the body as well as the already existing magnetic fields and electrical impulses. It can be used with other medication. Its essential purpose is to stabilise the magnetic and electrical forces in the body, which are often in a state of disarray considering modern man's lifestyle, stressors and a variety of other factors.

Magnets influence the whole body. But the blood in the body is most prone to this influence because of its iron content. Most of the iron in the body is in the blood. The remainder is in the muscles. As a result, the blood is immediately activated by the application of magnets. The process of ionisation is hastened, easing the free flow of blood throughout the body. This rejuvenates the system and activates the glands, regularising essential secretions.

The magnet also works on the other liquids and chemicals in the body. It reaches the magnetic fields within the body and works on the body internally. This also improves the generation of electrical impulses, and the entire body is activated.

7. Treatments for Specific Ailments

Magnetic polarity can be effectively used in a variety of ways to treat almost any problem. It is best used as an adjunct to aid the body in its healing process.

We shall now look at a variety of problems, which can be treated with magnetic polarity.

Treatment with magnets is simple, cheap and almost entirely free of side effects. Any ailment, condition or part of the body may be treated with magnets. Sometimes, the problem area can be treated directly. Specific glands or organs can also be treated. But remember, every body is unique and what works for one person may not work for another.

Also, magnets only help the body heal. So if a person is taking prescription medicines, s/he must not discontinue them without proper medical supervision. While the application of magnets to heal is not quackery by any yardstick, its scientific and proper use will depend on the therapist or physician who is using it as a medical aid. Self-help is best avoided and the application of magnets should always be under expert medical supervision.

We shall now look at a few diseases and their treatment with the application of magnets. We have also recommended the drinking of magnetised water to hasten the recovery process.

Aches, pains, strains, bruises and bone breaks are known to respond quickly to the application of magnets. Even the marks of bruises will go away if the site of the injury is treated with the North Pole immediately after injury. It is best to treat an injury with the North Pole until the pain and inflammation is gone.

After that, treating the same area with the south polarity will increase blood circulation, tissue oxygen saturation level and cell division rate. If there is bleeding, let it stop. Then if the North Pole is applied to the chest area, oxygen levels and blood circulation will increase.

In the case of fractures, the North Pole of a magnet, when placed on the upper portion of a crack, acts to soften and release calcium from the main bone. The South Pole of a similar magnet placed on the lower portion of the affected area draws fluid and calcium and directs them to where they are needed. Both the poles simultaneously applied speed up the healing process. Bipolar magnetised water can be drunk several times a day as an additional aid.

Injuries of all kinds are also helped by the application of magnets. If the injury is without any bleeding, apply the South Pole to eliminate pain and swelling. If there is any blood oozing from the injury, apply the north polarity on the point from where the blood is oozing. The north polarity can be applied on stitches too to hasten the healing of the cut. If the injury is long, both the poles can be applied together; the North Pole to the upper or right side and the South Pole to the lower or left side of the injury. The injury can be cleaned with magnetised water. Drinking magnetised water will also help.

There are different types of insects and so different types of bites, but the basic symptoms of itching, swelling and blisters are common. The north polarity should be applied on the bitten part immediately and the patient should be given magnetised water of the north polarity to drink.

Jaundice also reacts favourably to magnetic treatment. The North Pole of a medium-powered magnet should be applied under the right palm and the South Pole placed under the left palm for 10 minutes, both in the morning and in the evening. Bipolar magnetised water can be drunk several times a day. The South Pole of a medium-powered magnet should be applied on the liver. The treatment should continue for a few weeks.

Adrenal insufficiency can be treated by stimulation or sedation of the adrenal glands. This is only a temporary aid though. If strong magnets are used on any gland or organ it could result in overstimulation. Be careful of that. Overstimulation of any gland or organ is best avoided.

Arthritis is often helped by magnetic treatment. Magnets have been known to help stiffness in joints for centuries. Each person may need his or her own particular magnetic frequency and treatment time.

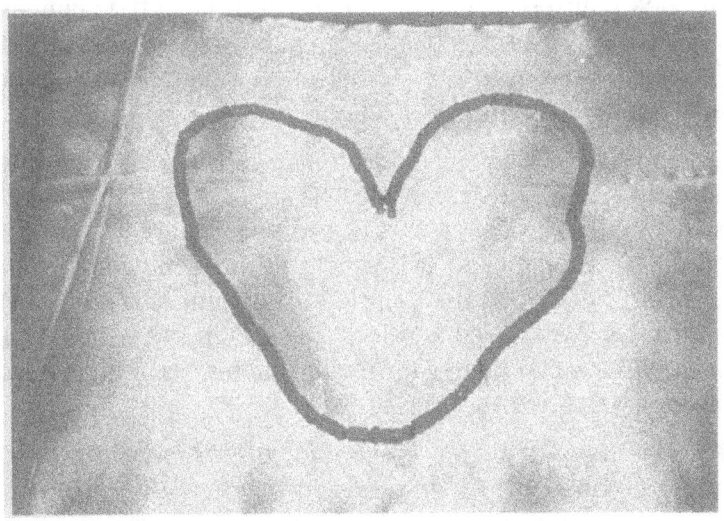

Magnet mala – meant to cure asthma, blood pressure and ailments of the lungs and spinal cord.

Asthma can be treated by placing the North Pole on the chest area. It is best to treat the problem as early as possible and also to treat the chest even when the individual is not having an attack. A pair of high-powered magnets should be applied under the palms for about 10 minutes in the morning and evening. The north polarity should be under the right palm and the south polarity under the left palm.

Crescent-type ceramic magnets also help the nose and throat. The north polarity should be applied on the right nostril and the south polarity on the left nostril covering the full nasal wall for about 10 minutes twice everyday. This will help with any difficulty in breathing. Crescent-type magnets can also be applied on the throat for about 10 minutes everyday. Magnetic necklaces are also helpful and can be worn throughout the day except while bathing.

Bipolar magnetised water of about two ounces each can be drunk several times a day. This helps clear any congestion in the lungs.

For back injuries, place magnets up and down the spine and even at the top of the head. Magnetic garments and belts with small disc magnets can be used effectively. Magnetic beds can also help back problems.

Backaches, which can include lumbago, spondylitis, rheumatic pain and slipped disc, can also be helped with magnets. If the pain is in the upper part of the body, the north polarity should be applied and if the pain is in the lower portion, the south polarity. If the pain is in the right side, the north polarity can be applied and if the pain is in the left side, the south polarity can be used. Bipolar magnetised water should also be consumed.

Magnets have also helped control grey hair. Both palms should be applied to high-powered magnets for 10 minutes in the morning and for the same period in the evening. Magnetised south polarity water should also be taken a few times a day. The treatment can be continued for months.

The common cold is also easily treated. The person suffering from it should keep both the palms on the centres of high-powered magnets for 10 minutes in the morning and 10 minutes in the evening. Crescent-type ceramic magnets should be applied on both the nostrils covering the nasal walls. Magnetised south polarity water should be taken regularly.

There are different types of cough and different reasons for it. But all coughs can be treated with high-powered magnets applied under the palms in the mornings and evenings. Crescent-type ceramic magnets can be applied on the throat several times of the day and night.

Diarrhoea and dysentery are treated in the same fashion. Appropriate magnets should be applied on the abdomen and also under the feet twice or thrice everyday. Bipolar magnetised water should be given after every stool or every two hours.

For ear pains, low potency crescent-type ceramic magnets are ideal. If there is pain in one ear only, the north polarity can be applied on the front of the ear and the south polarity on the back of the ear. If there is pain in both ears, the same treatment may be given to each ear one after the other. Medium-powered magnets can also be used if there are no results with ceramic magnets.

Eczema, herpes and ringworm can be treated with the north polarity. If there is any discharge, the magnet can be used over a tiny soft cloth placed on the discharge. This won't dirty the magnet. North polarity water can be drunk and the area affected washed with it as well.

Psoriasis has also been benefited by magnetic treatment. If the entire body has psoriasis, the north polarity of high-powered magnets may be applied under the right palm and the south polarity of the same magnet applied under the left palm. The same treatment should be carried out under the soles of the feet. North polarity magnetised water can be consumed several times a day.

In leucoderma, which is defective pigmentation of the skin, magnetic treatment helps cure small white patches of recent origin. If the patches are in the upper body, high-powered magnets can be applied under the palms and if the patches are in the lower body, magnets can be applied under the soles of the feet. Magnetised water should also be consumed at least a few times a day.

Some types of cancers have also been treated with magnets with favourable results. But only the North Pole should be applied at the site of the cancer as the South Pole can stimulate cancer cells and they may increase. Stimulating the thymus, which regulates the immune system, with the south polarity can help the body destroy cancer cells. Stimulating the liver may help rid the body of toxins. The south polarity helps increase blood flow and oxygen throughout the body, which will help the cells do their work. In life-threatening diseases like cancer, magnetic therapy can be useful along with any established medical treatment.

There have been many favourable reports of cancer treatment with magnets from different parts of the world. Experiments with mice and rabbits have also proved the efficacy of magnets against cancer.

In China, a magnetic bra has been developed with special, soft, flexible, magnetic bra inserts. Chinese physicians insist that the magnetic bra shrinks breast lumps without side effects.

The Carpal Tunnel Syndrome can be helped by wearing wristbands or wraps containing small magnets. There are several types of them with different magnetic configurations – north polarity towards the body, south polarity towards the body, and alternating them. The south polarity is good for prevention. For mild symptoms, alternating the magnetic forces will be fine. But if the condition is advanced with inflammation and pain, the north polarity may be necessary.

Constipation, if temporary, is an easy ailment to treat. Place a magnet of about 1,000 gauss over the colon with the stimulating polarity facing the body. The treatment may take just 15 minutes or less. The Japanese have developed a magnetic belt for constipation. It works with the south polarity and alternating polarity and has proved quite useful. The patient can also keep his right palm on the north polarity of a high-powered magnet. Simultaneously, his left sole should be on the South Pole. He should also drink magnetised bipolar water four to five times everyday. The treatment should be followed for a few months at least.

When there is a thickening of the cuticle or skin, it is called a corn. It is painful, compressed, thickened skin normally under and around the feet. High-powered or medium-powered magnets should be applied under the soles twice a day. North polarity magnetised water can be drunk, and the corns washed with it too.

Nose bleeds can have many causes. The patient should first be made to lie down with his head placed higher than the rest of the body. His nose should be plugged with cotton wool. High-powered magnets should be applied under the palms and crescent-type ceramic magnets should be applied on both the nostrils till the bleeding stops.

Eye diseases are of many kinds. In minor ailments, crescent-type ceramic magnets may be applied on both eyes even if the ailment affects only one eye. In serious cases, the South Pole of a high-powered magnet can be kept under the right palm for 10 minutes and the North Pole of a crescent-type ceramic magnet can be applied on each eye for five minutes along with a high-powered magnet. The eyes can also be washed with magnetised water of the north polarity. Magnetised water should also be drunk.

Trachoma is characterised by the formation of granules in the inner surface of the eyelids. It can spread to the cornea and even lead to blindness. The North Pole of crescent-type ceramic magnets should be applied on the affected eyes both morning and evening for about seven minutes each. The eyes should be washed with magnetised water of the north polarity, which can also be drunk.

For cataract, in which the lens of the eyes become opaque, magnetic therapy can help in the early stages. Crescent-type ceramic magnets can be applied on both eyes. High-powered magnets can also be applied under the palms. Magnetised water of the north polarity should be drunk and the eyes washed with it too.

In conjunctivitis, which is very common in Indian conditions, the eyes turn red, become painful and swollen and have a thick discharge. Magnetic treatment consists in applying both the poles of crescent-type ceramic magnets on both the eyes. The magnets should be applied several times a day and the eyes should be washed with magnetic water of the north polarity, which should also be drunk. Magnets can be applied under the palms too.

Fever is a symptom of many diseases. It is when the body raises its temperature to fight and kill germs. The magnetic treatment for all fevers is the same. Medium-powered magnets should be applied under the palms twice daily and magnetised bipolar water should be drunk every two hours.

Diabetes can be helped by placing a magnet over the pancreas for 30 minutes twice a day. This can stimulate the pancreas to produce more insulin. If the adrenal glands are overactive, application of the North Pole will bring their activity back to normal and help regulate blood sugar levels. Magnetic treatment works better with those who are not insulin dependent. The patient should keep his palms over high-powered magnets for 10 minutes in the morning. In chronic cases, the North Pole of a high-powered magnet should be applied on the pancreas and the South Pole on the back, opposite the pancreas. Bipolar magnetic water, taken a few times a day, strengthens the system.

Headaches are usually controlled well with magnets. The north polarity is generally recommended. Start early, at the first sign of pain. Stress headaches and headaches from eyestrain are usually relieved by North Pole treatment to the forehead. Migraine headaches may require treatment around the entire head area. Treatment, in this case, should be done even where there is no pain. Magnetic headbands are also commercially available now.

If the headache doesn't respond immediately, there may be other causes and other treatment sites. Liver or bowels can be checked. Crescent-type ceramic magnets should be applied on the forehead, between eyebrows or on both temples. A magnetic head belt can be tied on the forehead for 15 to 20 minutes once or twice a day.

In migraine a pair of crescent-type ceramic magnets or medium-powered magnets may be used. The North Pole should be applied on the right temple and the South Pole on the left temple. Regular intake of south polarity magnetised water and the use of a magnetic head belt also helps.

For mumps, crescent-type ceramic magnets may be applied to the area in pain for an hour or two in the mornings and evenings. The treatment should be given on both sides. The intake of north polarity magnetised water also helps.

Haemorrhoids can be treated with the north polarity, which is placed on the area. The length of treatment will depend on the severity of the case. Anyone suffering from fistula, fissures or piles should try and avoid being constipated, as it is the prime cause of the problem. Magnetic treatment for all these problems is the same. The patient should be asked to sit on the North and South Poles of a high-powered magnet for 10 minutes twice a day. He should drink magnetised water and wash the affected area with it.

Flatulence is the accumulation of wind in the bowels and can cause a lot of discomfort. High-powered magnets should be applied on both sides of the abdomen with the north polarity on the right side and the south polarity on the left side. South polarity magnetised water should be consumed. A magnetic stomach belt around the abdomen for an hour or two in the morning and evening also helps.

Hypertension is often caused by overactive adrenal glands. If that is the cause, magnets will help. For high blood pressure both the palms should be kept on two poles of high-powered magnets for about five minutes in the morning. It is the same treatment for low blood pressure but the magnet should be kept on for about 15 minutes. Magnetic wrist bands also help. The right wrist is ideal for high blood pressure and the left wrist for low blood pressure. The wristband should be kept for an hour at least. The drinking of bipolar magnetic water also helps regulate blood pressure.

Colic is a gripping pain in the colon. It can also be used to describe sharp, periodic pains in other organs. High- and medium-powered magnets can be used on the abdomen. The north polarity should be on the right side and the south polarity on the left side. Bipolar magnetised water also helps.

Insomnia can also be helped with the north polarity. A full-body magnetic pad or bed with the north polarity towards the body will help. The chest area can also be treated with north polarity for 15 minutes before going to sleep. Or the South Pole of a crescent-type ceramic magnet can be kept on the forehead between the eyebrows for 10 to 15 minutes before dozing off. The application of high-powered magnets under the palms and consuming south polarity magnetised water will also help.

Bead-size magnets can be taped on acupressure points to help reduce jet lag. The points (for the liver) are found between the big toe and the second toe, halfway towards the ankle. For the large intestine, the points are located in the middle of the webbed area between the thumb and the first finger. But if the magnets are on during sleep periods, the results may well be the opposite – you may be kept awake.

Infections in the kidneys are helped by the North Pole and sluggish action of the kidneys by the South Pole. Disc magnets can be worn for hours at a time. Large magnets can also be used for 15 to 30 minutes once or twice a day. There are different types of infections. They can include anuria or the suppression of urine, polyuria or increased urine output, haematuria or the passage of blood in the urine, renal colic or spasmodic pain radiating down the groin and retention of urine, which is simply the inability to pass urine. For all these conditions, high-powered magnets should be applied on the kidneys and the abdomen and also under the soles of the feet for half an hour in the mornings and evenings. Bipolar magnetised water should be drunk several times a day to flush the kidneys.

Nephritis or inflammation of the kidneys can be helped with the application of medium-powered magnets on the kidneys and high-powered magnets under the soles.

Magnetic treatment can help knees too. Knee pain is common in osteoarthritis, rheumatoid arthritis and gout. A nylon wrap, which contains many small magnets, is a helpful magnetic device. They are available in three types – with the magnets oriented north towards the body, with the south polarity towards the body or alternating both north and south polarities. One of them is bound to work depending on the problem. The North Pole of high-powered magnets should be kept over the affected side of the right knee and the South Pole on the affected left knee for about 10 minutes in the morning. In the evening, both the soles may be kept on both the magnets. Bipolar magnetised water can be consumed several times a day. If there is localised pain in any knee, the South Pole of a crescent-type ceramic magnet can be tied over the spot for several hours in the night.

In rheumatism, high-powered magnets should be applied under the palms if the problem is primarily in the upper part of the body. Magnets can be applied under the soles of the feet if the problem is centred on the lower part of the body. If the knees are affected, both magnets should be applied on the knees, the North Pole on the right knee and the South Pole on the left knee. South polarity magnetised water should be consumed at regular intervals.

In sciatica, there can be intense pain in either leg or both the legs. The North Pole of high-powered magnets should be applied on the hip from where the pain starts and the South Pole should be placed under the sole of the affected leg. South polarity magnetised water should be consumed. It is a long treatment process.

In sinusitis, high-powered magnets should be applied under the palms and crescent-type ceramic magnets on both sides of the nose or over the eyebrows, depending on the area of pain. Magnetic foils or other small magnets can be applied directly over sinuses. The direct application of magnets on the area works, but the effects are temporary. The endocrine system and the kidneys will also have to be looked into for possible causes and given the right polarity to hasten the healing process.

A clogged liver can be stimulated with the south polarity and an infected liver with the north polarity. It would be better to use a large area magnet for up to an hour once or twice a day. Liver enlargement is also a common condition. The North Pole of high-powered magnets should be applied on the painful and swollen part of the liver, and the South Pole on the back just opposite the North Pole. Bipolar magnetised water drunk a few times a day also helps.

Lumbago is pain in the lower portion of the back in the lumbar region. High-powered magnets must be applied on the painful part. If the pain is on the upper and lower parts of the spinal cord, apply the North Pole on the upper side and the South Pole on the lower side. If the pain is horizontal, the North Pole should be applied on the right side and the South Pole on the left side. Magnetised south polarity water should be drunk several times a day.

For loss of memory, high-powered magnets should be applied to the palms in the morning and to the soles in the evening. South polarity magnetised water should be drunk a few times a day.

Magnetic therapy has also helped in the treatment of multiple sclerosis. The stimulating south polarity can be applied to the entire spine and the base of the head. For cases that are not too severe, permanent magnets of the right polarity can be worn for many hours a day with beneficial results.

Neck and shoulder pains are greatly helped by wearing magnetic necklaces. These necklaces have been in use for hundreds of years and are quite useful. They can be decorative too. They are in vogue now as modern lifestyles contribute heavily to neck, shoulder and spinal pains. Because they are decorative, these necklaces have also become a fashion statement in addition to being a valuable treatment option.

Spondylitis is fairly common these days. It is the inflammation of the vertebrae of the spine. There are different types of spondylitis. The condition is very painful and disabling. Magnetic treatment helps. If X-rays reveal that any vertebra has slipped from its position, the North Pole of a high-powered magnet helps bring it back to position. The South Pole of a similar magnet should be placed on the point where the pain begins.

The use of magnetic fields after surgery can help speed the healing process and reduce scar tissue. The north polarity helps pain and inflammation and the south polarity helps heal. This technique is also good for minor wounds and cuts.

The problem of excess weight can also be treated with magnets. Magnetic earrings help stimulate relevant points in the ear which suppress appetite. So if overeating is a problem, this is a quick solution. North polarity magnets can also be placed over fatty areas and stronger magnets can be placed over larger fat deposits to reduce their concentration. The right palm should be kept on the North Pole and the left palm on the South Pole of high-powered magnets in the morning for 10 to 15 minutes.

The same treatment can be continued in the evening under the soles of the feet. Bipolar magnetised water can be taken several times a day. Magnets can also be applied on heavy hips, abdomen and other areas of fat accumulation.

Magnetic treatment has also helped facial paralysis. Medium-powered or crescent-type ceramic magnets can be applied to the affected part. The North Pole can be applied to the upper part and the South Pole to the lower part. The consumption of south polarity magnetised water also helps.

For pneumonia, appropriate magnets can be applied under the palms and bipolar magnetised water should be drunk every few hours.

The pancreas can also be stimulated with the south polarity if they are sluggish. This gland is located one inch above and left of the navel. Small disc magnets can be placed inside and outside clothing to hold each other. They can be worn comfortably for hours.

Prostrate enlargement can be treated with daily application of an hour or two of the north polarity. Sitting on the magnetic power pad is reasonably comfortable. Tumours should not be treated with the south polarity because it stimulates cell growth and, in this case, can stimulate the growth of malignant cells. High-powered magnets can be applied on both ends of the enlarged prostate. This can be done even thrice a day for difficult cases. South polarity magnetised water will help the passage of urine.

Magnets can also reduce stress. Magnetic treatments are easily applied to back, neck, knees, chest, eyes and other parts to help the body relax. The North Pole will reduce specific aches and pains and the South Pole will strengthen the body to counteract the effects of stress.

Tooth problems can also be helped by magnetic treatment. The north polarity is good for inflammation and infection and the south polarity is strengthening. A magnetic brush is available these days. There are two small magnets in the head of the brush with the North Pole towards the bristles. Apparently those who have used the magnetic brush say it works well.

Magnets can also be used effectively for a number of children's diseases. Ulcers in the mouth or Apthae are painful and may sometimes bleed. Since this problem is essentially caused by bad digestion, appropriate magnets should be placed under the palms and low-powered magnets applied on the cheeks. North polarity magnetised water should be drunk several times a day.

Ulcers improve when the north polarity is applied directly on the area. Drinking magnetically treated water has also helped. Overactive adrenal glands can also cause ulcers and may need to be looked at and given the necessary magnetic polarity.

Bed-wetting is a common condition with children but if it continues after the age of four, it should be treated. Appropriate magnets should be applied under the soles of children before they go to sleep for about ten minutes. Magnets can also be placed on both sides of the bladder.

Polio is still prevalent in India despite massive efforts by the government. A child afflicted with it is crippled for life. For children above two years of age, the North Pole of medium-powered magnets can be applied on the hip of the side affected and the South Pole kept below the sole of the affected side. If both the legs are affected, the right leg may be treated in the morning and the left leg in the evening.

They can also be treated on alternate days. Children below the age of two can be treated with ceramic-type magnets. Bipolar magnetised water should be consumed several times a day.

Worms of all kinds are another common problem. After confirming the diagnosis with a stool test, magnetic treatment should be given by applying magnets of appropriate strength under the soles of the child, preferably in the evening. North polarity magnetised water should be consumed several times a day.

Dentition troubles are also common among children. Small magnets should be placed in the fists of the child and s/he should be made to drink bipolar magnetised water.

Mental retardation in children is also helped with magnetotherapy. Medium- or high-powered magnets, depending on the situation, should be applied under the palms in the morning and under the soles in the evening. Bipolar magnetised water should be consumed several times a day.

Heart diseases are increasingly common now. Magnetic treatment can help. The right palm should be kept on the North Pole and the left palm on the South Pole of high-powered magnets for about five minutes a day. It can be increased to about ten minutes slowly and should be done in the mornings. South polarity magnetised water should be drunk a few times everyday.

Strange, but true. It works. Magnets can help a person increase height! The idea is to stimulate the pituitary gland. The North Pole of a crescent-type ceramic magnet should be applied to the centre of the forehead between the eyebrows, above the upper portion of the nose. The South Pole of a similar magnet should be placed just opposite the North Pole for about ten minutes every morning.

The next day the North Pole magnet may be shifted to between the right ear and the head and the South Pole magnet to between the left ear and the head. Alternate this treatment every day. South polarity magnetised water should be drunk thrice a day at least. This treatment should be continued for months. The change in height can then be measured.

Hernia is the protrusion of the intestine from its normal position. It can be very painful. If the hernia is on both sides, the North Pole of a high-powered magnet may be applied on the right side and the south polarity applied on the left side. If the hernia is only on one side, placing the North Pole on the front and the South Pole on the back, opposite the North Pole, is ideal. South polarity magnetised water can be drunk several times a day. When hernia occurs in children, the strength of the magnet can be selected according to their age.

When fluid accumulates in large amounts around the testicles, it is known as hydrocele. High-powered magnets should be applied under the soles and the South Pole of a crescent-type magnet should be applied to the swollen testicle. It is a long treatment.

Magnets also help strengthen the nervous system. Both the North and South Poles of a high-powered magnet should be applied under the palms in the morning and under the soles in the evening. Bipolar magnetised water should be consumed many times a day. The treatment should be continued for a long time to ensure that the nerves are strengthened and remain strengthened.

In neuralgia, there is pain in the nerves and in neuritis the nerves are inflamed. The treatment for both is the same. If the pain is vertical, the north polarity should be applied on the upper end and the south polarity on the lower end. If the pain is horizontal, apply the North Pole on the right side and the South Pole on the left side of the stretch. South polarity magnetised water can be drunk several times a day.

Gonorrhoea is a sexually transmitted disease and if left untreated can affect the vital organs. The North Pole of a high-powered magnet should be applied under the soles of both feet, one after the other, for 15 minutes each in the morning and evening. The North Pole of medium-powered magnets should be applied on both sides of the area of pain or the North Pole of a crescent-type magnet can be tied to the spot at night. North polarity magnetised water should be drunk and the area washed with it.

Amenorrhoea is the medical term for scanty menstruation. It can have many causes. Two high-powered magnets should be kept next to one another and the patient asked to sit on them for about half an hour every day for a few weeks. Bipolar magnetised water should be drunk several times a day. It is the same treatment for dysmenorrhoea or painful menstruation, menopausal problems, menorrhagia or excessive menstrual bleeding and metorrhagia or uterine haemorrhage.

Leucorrhoea is an excess of sticky, white, offensive discharge from the vagina. It can be a difficult problem but the timely use of magnets can help. It also follows the same treatment procedure.

Cracked nipples are also helped by magnets. Medium-powered magnets can be held on the nipples or crescent-type ceramic magnets can be softly tied on them. If there are cracks only on one nipple, the North Pole can be applied to it. North polarity magnetised water should be consumed and the nipples washed with it.

Tumours in the uterus can also be treated with high-powered magnets placed on the uterus on the front and the South Pole on the back, opposite the North Pole. Malignant tumours should be treated only with the North Pole and north polarity magnetised water should be drunk.

8. Some More Research and Treatments

Studies have shown that magnetically treated water increases plant growth. It was found that plants watered only with magnetically treated South Pole water increased their growth compared to plants watered with tap water.

Conversely, plants watered with North Pole treated water grew at a much slower pace. Also, freshly-cut roses placed on north polarity magnets lasted longer while the south polarity made them lose their petals. Even sprouts watered with south polarity grew more abundantly. These findings are significant because it conclusively proves that magnets affect all life forms.

Enormous research has also been done with water. Water crystals are known to take different shapes and forms depending on the environment in which they are formed. Music, the spiritual, emotional and physical energy of the place, its history, epidemics, the mood of the people and several other factors influence the formation of water crystals. There are 'healthy' and 'unhealthy' crystals and the consumption of 'unhealthy' crystallised water can endanger the health of the people in that area.

Japanese scientists have conclusively proved that water crystals can even be moody – they can smile and be sad! When over 70 per cent of the body is liquid, any such finding is of enormous importance in the understanding of the human body and in the treatment of disease.

Water can form nine different three-dimensional structures. Magnetic forces apparently influence the kind of structures that are formed. Kirlian photographs of magnetically-treated water showed that it was apparently more organised by the application of magnetic forces. Besides water, juices, wine, beer and milk can also be treated with magnets. In fact, any liquid can be treated with magnets.

In an experiment in Tokyo University, mice were kept in a magnetic force of 4,200 gauss for 59 days. After they were removed from the magnetic field, the average life-span of their red blood cells increased from 70 to over 100 days. The mice also managed to live a third longer than their average life-span.

Experiments with magnets have also been done on chickens, worms and other animals. Positive results have also been noted in plants, in their seed yield, vitality and growth. Biological activity is certainly enhanced by magnets of the proper polarity.

It has been observed that living organisms often suffer when there is a fall in the magnetic force of the earth. Birds become less active and their egg-laying capacity reduces. The longer an organism is deprived of magnetism, the less fertile it becomes. It also has a shorter life-span. Plants and other small organisms, including tadpoles, grew faster and bigger when magnetically treated.

Experiments have proved that all life is touched by magnetic forces in the cosmos. To give a simplistic example, even the electrical and magnetic emissions from a television set can affect the human body. Even electric poles close to a house can affect the residents. Enormous electrical discharges can result in symptoms commonly associated with chronic fatigue syndrome. Even Vaastu and Feng Shui, the traditional Oriental concepts of health, well-being and happiness, mention this in no uncertain terms.

Many experiments have also been conducted on human beings. It has been seen that wrinkles have diminished when magnetic treatments have been combined with the application of a cream. Experiments have also shown that elderly people treated with electromagnets found their hair getting darker. They even became more energetic.

Magnetic fields also hasten wound healing and reduce the formation of scar tissue. Pulsed magnetic fields of the proper strength and frequency have been found to affect each major atomic element in the body. As biophysicists further discover the molecules involved in ageing, magnetic treatments might be used to restart, stimulate or unlock the ageing keys. Research into the use of magnets has gained a sophistry and pace only in recent times. In the coming years, there is little doubt that when more is known about magnets and their influence on all life forms, the use of magnets may well become a way of life.

Burl Payne, a practitioner of magneto-therapy in the United States, has conducted several experiments with magnets. This experiment may explain a point. He took a bunch of grapes from the same stalk, washed and separated them into two groups of about 20 grapes each. He placed them in identical bowls, one over the north polarity and the other over the south polarity. There was a perceptible difference in taste in a few minutes. Soon it was evident that the grapes treated with the south polarity were much sweeter than the grapes treated with the north polarity.

Payne reversed the polarities and the grapes started tasting different, again within minutes! The less tasty grapes were sweet now and the sweet grapes had reduced sweetness.

A simple experiment. As simple as it can get. Yet, the results are amazing in their significance. If a bunch of grapes can be influenced by magnetic polarities in such a short time, one can well imagine the influence of magnets on the larger scheme of life.

Payne repeated the experiments with oranges, strawberries and other fruits with similar results. Even frozen juices improved their taste when treated with the south polarity.

The world has understood the power of magnetic healing but continuous research is underway and necessary to determine the precise mechanism by which pulsed magnetic fields aid healing. Research continues to determine the optimum pulse rates, waveforms and amplitudes to use in treatment. Effective treatment times need to be determined and it has to be understood if magnetic forces produce actual regeneration of damaged tissue or whether there is only temporary improvement.

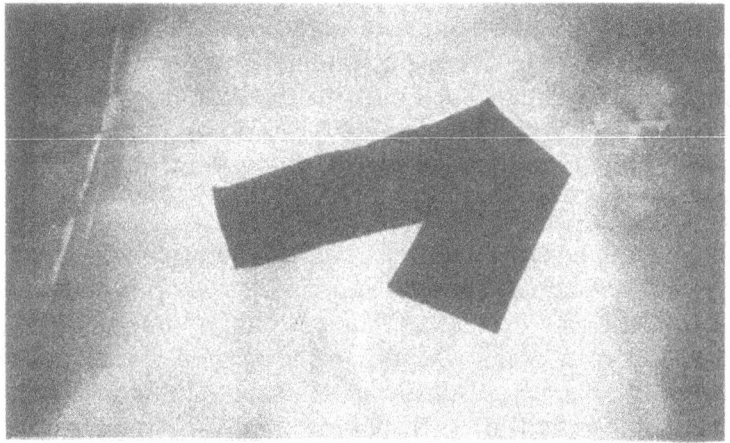

Wristband – used for blood pressure and arthritic pain in the hands.

In 1976, a Japanese physician carried out a large study on more than 11,000 people with symptoms of stiff necks, painful muscles, rheumatism and neuralgia. The north polarity was pointed to the body and the magnets were applied to specific acupressure points. More than 90 per cent of the patients said the treatment was effective.

A second Japanese study used magnetic necklaces with both poles sideways to the skin. Most patients reported pain relief. This study is significant because it suggests that the use of simultaneous magnetic polarities is not as effective as the use of the appropriate single pole.

In March 1984, the prestigious British medical journal The Lancet, which is not wont to encourage quackery or anything even remotely associated with it, published an article on the results of pulsed magnetic forces on persistent rotator cuff tendonitis or shoulder pains. This mention is far-reaching because The Lancet believes thorough scientific research is the only paradigm for a mention in its pages. This definitely gave magneto-therapy a fillip.

A group of patients who didn't respond to the conventional corticosteroid injections showed considerable improvement after being treated with magnets. What is more, no side effects were noticed.

When magnets are applied to the body, the blood flow increases and the oxygen absorbed by the tissues also increases. Studies have shown up to a 200 per cent increase in dissolved oxygen in the tissues. Research on how magnetic forces alter the change in blood cells continues.

The most conclusive results with magnets is in the treatment of arthritis. In controlled experiments all over the world, different types of arthritis were successfully treated by pulsed magnetic forces with no side effects at all. In a preliminary study on rats, in whom arthritis was artificially produced, the inflammation could be got rid of in three or four days using pulsed magnetic forces.

Evidently, magnets are a powerful healing tool. However, each person may need his or her own particular magnetic frequency to be determined for quick and precision healing.

9. Duration of Treatment

Treatments of 15 to 30 minutes twice a day are sufficient for most conditions if pulsed magnetic forces are used; half an hour to several days if permanent magnets are used; or up to 30 days or more if magnetic flex pads or magnetic foils are used.

But the real judge of the treatment is the patient. Body wisdom should be respected. The part of the body being treated will send signals if the treatment is continued past the optimum time. Listen to the body, use magnets, if necessary, as an accessory to conventional treatment, and be prepared to make changes in its use as the situation demands.

For acute conditions, improvement may be observed in as little as a few minutes. If there is no improvement at all, which can happen sometimes, then continued magnetic treatment probably will not help. Drop it.

In the case of chronic or long-term ailments, the results will quite naturally take longer. Many conditions, like the patient's general health, are important. Results may be evident only after a month or more of daily treatments.

Remember, magnets don't heal; they help the body heal. So to prevent a recurrence of the problem, it is also necessary to adopt the right habits like a good diet, a positive attitude and sufficient exercise. The preventive use of magnets can also be adopted once the person gets well.

Magneto-therapists all over the world have reported amazing results with magnets for nearly all diseases. But there are many variables at play like different constitutions, temperaments, dietary habits, climate, age, the type of disease, how chronic it is, hereditary factors, lifestyle, habits and so on.

There is no fixed rule on how long a cure will take. A magnet is normally applied only once a day but in chronic cases it may have to be applied twice a day. In the beginning, to gauge susceptibility to magnetic effect, a magnet should be applied for not more than five minutes. Children should never be exposed to strong magnets. The total time a magnet is used can be raised to 20 or 30 minutes twice a day but that will depend on the disease and the tolerance of the patient.

Even after achieving a cure, the magnets should be used for regaining strength. Healthy patients can use a magnet for 10 minutes a day as a preventive.

How Safe are the Treatments?

In 1994, four physicians published an article in the Journal of Rheumatology on the value of pulsed magnetic fields for treating arthritis. They stated that over 200,000 patients had been safely treated with pulsed magnetic forces without toxic side effects.

Two Chinese physicians and acupuncturists, Hsu and Fong, reported in a 1978 American Journal of Acupuncture article, "From an experience of several tens of thousands of cases covering nearly one hundred types of complaints, no contraindications have been found."

Apparently, there are no side effects.

But the improper use of magnets can interfere with body chemistry. Nausea, headache or irritability can be temporarily produced by using the wrong polarity or too strong a magnet. It is best to let the body talk.

Magnets work by acting on the atomic constitution of cells forming blood and other chemical fluids as well as on the magnetic fields already existing inside the body. The magnetic effect does bring about certain modifications in body fluids and can sometimes cause reactions, especially when strong magnets are applied. People can experience different feelings ranging from heaviness in the head to heavy perspiration to dryness in the tongue or even giddiness.

But these reactions are short-lived and not dangerous at all. So there is no need to panic.

Precautions

All bio-magnetic aids should be kept away from fire. The patient should desist from cold drinks and food for an hour after the use of belly and knee belts. Bath should also be abstained from for an hour after the use of magnets.

1. Choice of Magnets

Magnets are available in all shapes, sizes and powers. Now the choice of magnet to be used rests solely with the magneto-therapist. Disc-shaped magnets are ideal for the palms, soles and the torso. But for uneven parts like the forehead, eyes, ears, nose, cheeks and throat, crescent-shaped magnets are the best.

Both the poles of a magnet have to be applied individually and usually concurrently. So two magnets of the same size and strength are needed. Normally stronger shaped-disc magnets are used on palms, soles and limbs while weak ceramic magnets should be applied only to the head, face, chest and wrist. The bands, chains and necklaces are usually for longer and more constant use and so are fitted with weak and small magnets.

Types of Permanent Magnets

There are many types of artificial magnets. There is the soft iron variety, which is the first type of permanent magnet made. It is much stronger than natural lodestone. But pure iron doesn't stay magnetised for long.

Alnico is the first type of alloyed magnetic material. It is made by mixing nickel and aluminium with iron.

In the ceramic variety, barium ferrite magnets have been manufactured in the United States since 1954. Barium combines with iron atoms to form barium ferrite. It can be powdered, melted and cast into any desired shape or size and then magnetised.

Rubber magnets are of a flexible plastic material mixed with powdered barium ferrite to produce a material that is fairly strong magnetically. It is usually magnetised in strips of alternating polarity.

Strontium also combines chemically with iron to form a magnetic compound. It can also be powdered and cast into different shapes.

Among the rare earth magnets, samarium and cobalt can be mixed with pure iron to produce a very strong magnetic material, which can be made in small sizes too.

The most recently discovered and most powerful type of magnet material is made by combining the rare earth element neodymium with iron and a little boron. This can be cast and shaped in small sizes.

A wide range of magnetic materials is available today. There are tiny magnets the size of buttons, domino-size ceramic magnets, cookie-size disc magnets, rectangular block magnets and bar magnets almost an inch thick.

Magnets may have one pole on each end or face, or the poles may alternate across a face. When magnetic powder is embedded in plastic, it can be made into any number of shapes. They can be mounted in bandages, tapes, vests and shoe inserts or they can be strung on a necklace, made into a bracelet, or used to cover a whole mattress.

There are several kinds of permanent magnets. Alnico was the first type of magnetic alloy manufactured. Today, ferrite or ceramic magnets are very common. Ferrites can be powdered and cast into any shape or mixed with flexible plastic to produce magnetic strips or sheets.

Normally magnets with the poles on the large faces are required and not on the ends because the face with the correct polarity has to be laid against the body of the person being treated. The most inexpensive way to do home treatment is usually with permanent magnets. If there is a large area to treat, pulsed magnetic healing devices may be cheaper and more effective.

Let us now take a look at different types of magnets in use for therapeutic purposes.

Magnetic Beads

These are tiny magnets which are taped over acupuncture points.

Magnetic Beds

There are several varieties of magnetic beds in vogue all over the world. They consist of magnets embedded in pads that one sleeps on. Designers have now added crystals, copper wire designs, mineral mixtures and other materials and devices to magnetic beds. Magnetic beds have made inroads all over the world, thanks to modern marketing techniques. Many 'magnet' millionaires and 'magnet' healthy people have since been born.

Block Magnets

These are fairly large with gauss strength of one thousand. They can be used for short periods.

Magnetic Bracelets

These have also caught on all over the world. They have been found to relieve stress and minor ailments like arthritis, nervous disorders and insomnia as well as improving the circulation and health of the muscular system. They are also easily available in department stores and by mail order.

Disc Magnets

Without holes in the centre, they are available in diameters of two inches and less. Flat discs are handy for treating minor aches and pains. They can be applied in pairs. One can be placed inside a garment and one outside to hold each other in place. They are very convenient and can even pass off for the latest in sartorial elegance.

Magnetic Foils
With alternating magnetic polarities, they are inexpensive, easy to apply to the body and effective in relieving pain.

Magnetic Garments
Magnets have now been added to a variety of garments. But the polarity and weight of the magnet should be considered. For example, bras should have the North Pole towards the body to discourage the growth of tumours.

When stitched to garments, there is a good chance that the polarity may get switched and that may not be beneficial. So extra care should be taken to stitch the magnet in the right direction with as much care as possible.

Magnetic Power Pads
They are quite powerful and useful for treating water, sweetening fruit and placing on different parts of the body.

Magnetic Necklaces
Like bracelets, necklaces have become major adornments. They have dual roles now, especially as they are marketed as healing tools. Magnetic necklaces were first reported to be used by a French physician in 400 AD. In those days they must have been heavy, bulky and crude and made out of lodestones. Now there are beautiful necklaces: lightweight, high-gauss necklaces from samarium-cobalt-iron alloys. Another attractive necklace is made from hematite, a shiny grey-black iron ore.

A necklace can be wrapped around the head to prevent a headache. It can be worn around a wrist, elbow, knee, foot or hand. It can even be placed over the eyes to give them a soothing magnetic rejuvenation. They are also good for stiff necks and sore shoulders.

They can be worn throughout the day and night except while bathing.

Magnetic Belts

The head belt can be worn or tied around the forehead for 15 to 30 minutes at a time or twice a day. It helps relieve headache, migraine and other problems.

The throat belt can be worn or tied around the neck for about 15 to 30 minutes at a time once or twice daily. It helps treat cough, tonsillitis and other similar complaints of the throat.

The blood pressure belt can be worn on the right wrist for those with high blood pressure and on the left wrist for those with low blood pressure. It can be worn for two to three hours a day.

The belly belt is specially designed for problems of the abdomen and the back. It helps in cases of colitis, hernia, prostrate problems and other similar conditions. It can be used twice a day for an hour or two at each sitting.

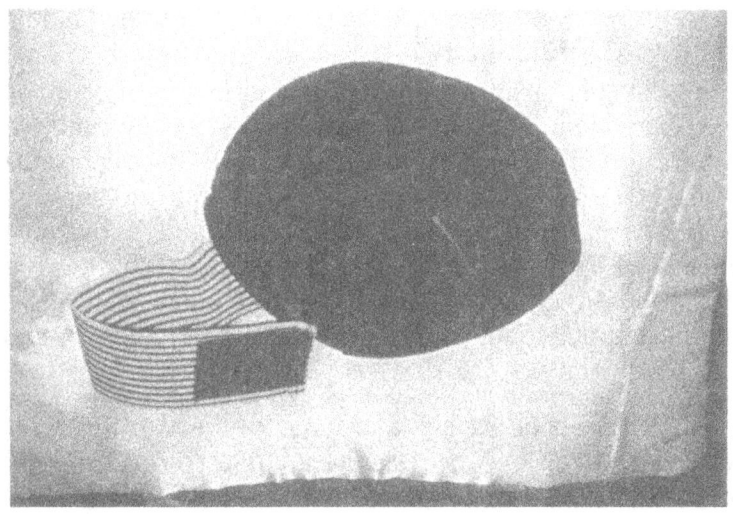

Knee belt – relieves pain in the knees, elbows and shoulder bone.

The knee belt can be tied to the affected knee for an hour or two once or twice everyday. It helps with muscular pains, swellings in the knee joints, arthritis and other problems. It is also easy and convenient to use. It can be tied on one knee and then the other knee. Two belts can also be used simultaneously on both knees.

Magnetisation of Water

We have already talked about the effect of magnets on all life forms including liquids. The drinking of magnetised water, along with magnetic treatment, is recommended by most magneto-therapists. It forms a complete treatment. Magnetised water can also be consumed as a preventive as well as a post-treatment maintenance regimen.

When water or any liquid is kept in contact with a permanent magnet for a certain period, its magnetism passes into it. Water can be magnetised in different ways.

One method is to suspend a magnet over an empty pot. Water is poured over the magnet in a thin stream, which is collected in the pot. This has its drawbacks though and is not a recommended method.

The other method is to place a magnet for a few hours in a pot filled with water. The water slowly gets magnetised. This method has many limitations too.

The third method, which is the best, is to fill the water in two tumblers or any containers with flat bottoms. One container should be put on the centre of one magnet in which the North Pole is exposed and the other container should be placed on another container in which the South Pole is exposed. The magnets should be disc type, round and flat, with a diameter of about 10 cms. The bottoms of the containers should cover the surfaces of the magnets used. The containers should be of glass, stainless steel or plastic.

This will help the free flow of magnetism. The containers can be kept on the magnets for many hours. After the containers are taken off the magnets, the water from both containers can be mixed or kept separately. If the water is mixed, it becomes bipolar water. If it isn't, it can be used separately as North Pole and South Pole water.

When water is magnetised, the degree of magnetisation and the therapeutic utility of bipolar and unipolar magnetism needs to be studied. The degree of magnetisation depends on the quantity of water used, the power of the magnet and the duration of contact. While the power of magnets can be measured, there is no method to measure the degree of magnetisation of water.

Magnetised water is often prescribed as an addition to magnetic treatment. Different magneto-therapists use different doses for different treatments. There is no standard gauge and the modalities will depend on the therapist, the ailment and the patient.

After a great deal of experimentation, Dr Samuel Hahnemann came up with three homeopathic medicines. One was from the combination of both the North and the South Pole, and the other two were from the two poles each. He laid down precise symptoms for the use of these three medicines. Normally, only bipolar water is prescribed. But there is no doubt that the treatment will be more specific if the other poles are also used independently.

Apart from water, other liquids can also be magnetised and with good results too. If milk is kept on the South Pole for about half an hour and then ingested every day it is an excellent remedy for exhaustion. Fruit juices and even beer have benefited with magnetisation. Magnetised medicinal oils have been particularly useful in the treatment of rheumatism.

Magnetised water regulates bowel movements and rids the body of toxins. It can be used as a preventive by healthy persons too. Water kept in a magnetised container for about six hours can be consumed every day. It also helps with blood pressure problems, normalises the circulatory system and helps in clearing clogged arteries. It is also useful in the treatment of asthma, bronchitis and coughs and colds.

Magnetised water can also be used for washing swollen, sore and tired eyes, wounds and some skin diseases. Regular washing of the eyes with magnetised water is an excellent preventive care.

The Spin Force

There is a biological force around the human body that appears to be a special type of spin force. It presumably exists around all living things. It is virtually everywhere. This force is not magnetic but its amplitude varies with changes in the earth's magnetic field.

This force causes hanging objects to rotate around the body. It usually moves in a clockwise direction and varies with the emotional state or vitality of the person. This force is estimated to be over one million times as large as the body's magnetic field. This force may be related to what is normally known as chi, prana, life force or the other names given to it in different cultures. This spin force is an entirely different kind of force. Magnetism may only be a lower order of the spin force.

Based on this discovery, spin may be considered a fundamental force along with the other fundamental forces. To quote Burl Payne, who has experimented a lot with the spin force and from whose substantial works on the application of magnets we have borrowed for the benefit of readers, "Spin is everywhere, around every object in the universe. Each force subsumes the lower one. Spin forces produce rotation, magnetic forces twist, push and pull, electric ones push or pull and gravity only pulls. In this way, the forces help to structure the universe. If magnetic forces weren't operating, electrons and protons would eventually find one another and annihilate in a flash of light. If there were no spin forces, gravity would eventually draw everything together. Spin is the complement to gravity, keeping particles orbiting around whether or not they are electrically charged."

Burl Payne points out that the spin force related to magnetism is not in the same direction as the spin force that makes planets and stars spin around their axes.

More research is required in this area, of course, but one shouldn't block out the fact that there are different types of magnetism. Electron spin resonance is a field of study that involves changing electron spins by the application of magnetic forces. Nuclear Magnetic Resonance Imaging, which uses changes in proton spins, is also a big field of study and more research into these areas will help understand how magnetic forces really heal.

Cancer Cure and More Research

The future is truly magnetic if one were to examine the enormous potential of magneto-therapy and the pace of accelerated research into the subject. The recent invention of a super-magnet (NaturChem's Zinc-coated Super Health Magnets) with great strength and a minute size has far-reaching significance. These super-magnets were allegedly used with great success on breast cancer patients and promise to revolutionise the treatment of cancer.

The super-energy permanent magnet used in the treatment had a maximum energy product of up to 36,000,000 gauss-oersteds.

According to the prestigious American Journal of Science (1990), the strength of the super-magnet was a world record in commercial production. The super-magnet was invented in 1983 and is now getting global recognition. William Philpott, MD, a well-known medical researcher, has written about it in his new book, Biomagnetic Handbook: Guide to Medical Magnets, The Energy Medication of Tomorrow, New Hope for Physical & Emotional Illness. The super-magnet used in the cancer treatment resembled an American quarter in size and weighed 30 grams.

Each one of the three women with breast cancer had a super-magnet hanging around her neck for about four months, with the north polarity of the magnet directed towards the body. This is important: if the super-magnet had been placed directly on the tumour, as conventional magnetic treatment would suggest, the results would have followed expected lines. But since the super-magnet hung around the neck of each cancer patient, it can safely be assumed that they influenced the entire body.

It is also important to note that healthy tissue surrounding the tumour was not harmed by the super-magnet. The researchers believe that the mechanism at play, when the super-magnet is trying to eliminate a malignant tumour, is based on Wollin's discovery of a universal spiral theory, quite similar to Burl Payne's theory.

Wollin, a researcher, discovered that spirals are found throughout nature, right from the galaxies, each one consisting of hundreds of billions of stars, down to the basic shape of DNA (deoxyribonucleic acid) – the body's ultimate genetic material, the miraculous molecule that makes a mouse a mouse or a human being a human being. DNA exists in every chromosome in every cell of every individual.

The researchers believe that magnetism and cancer cells are spirals on different scales. When super-magnetism is applied to cancer tumours, the magnetic spirals, being larger, dominate, and finally kill the smaller cancer cell spirals.

The researchers insist that the successful results of the cancer treatment project are a logical consequence of more than 400 years of research in the field of electromagneto-therapy and diseases.

Electromagneto-therapy has a long history. From Paracelsus, one of the greatest physicians of the Middle Ages (he died in 1541), to Professor Bjorn Nordenstrom, a radiologist at the Karolinska Hospital in Stockholm. Evidently, research into the subject has been very profound.

In a book chapter entitled About Magnets and Their Wonderful Ability to Help in the Cure of All Sorts of Diseases by Paracelsus, he writes, for example, that he found the use of magnets to be of great value in the treatment and cure of epilepsy. He recommends that four magnets be placed on the stomach and four on the back.

Bjorn Nordenstrom has also treated breast and lung cancer tumour patients with electromagneto-therapy. His treatment reportedly regressed or killed tumours in most of the 80 patients.

Nordenstrom's treatment of malignant tumours consists in inserting a long needle into the centre of a tumour and another needle into normal tissue. The needles are platinum electrodes. The electrode in the tumour is positive and the other negative. Wires are hooked to both electrodes and connected to a direct electric current processor. The electric current is turned on and is increased in successions from 0 to 10 volts, creating an electromagnetic field.

Two doctors, Gosta Wollin and Eric Enby, believe they have developed a new method for curing cancer. They feel that the successful use of only one magnet was possible because a human being is like a magnet. There is enough evidence to prove this.

That humans are electromagnetic was suggested in 1926 by the eminent American surgeon and electromagnet therapist George Crile in his book Bipolar Theory of Living Processes and by the eminent radiologist and cancer researcher Bjorn Nordenstrom, in 1983, in his book Biological Electric Circuits: Clinical, Experimental and Theoretical Evidence for an Additional Circular System.

The doctors are continuing with their clinical research on the treatment of cancer because this could well be one of the greatest medical breakthroughs in recent times.

The incidence of cancer worldwide is rising at an alarming rate. Normally, when someone has cancer, there are three ways of trying to eliminate the malignant tumour from the body. Surgery is one possibility. Another possibility is to kill the cancerous cells with radiation or radiotherapy, which, of course, is also electromagneto-therapy. The third option is to kill the cancerous cells with drugs, that is, chemotherapy. The drawback with these treatments is that they can damage healthy cells too.

The new option is the use of electromagneto-therapy with the employment of super-magnets. This treatment does not damage healthy cells because healthy cells have different electromagnetic potential than cancer cells.

It is also inexpensive and a more humane approach.

The Beginning of Modern Research

Dr Philpott, who has co-authored Brain Allergies: The Psycho-Nutrient Connection, Victory Over Diabetes: A Bio-Ecologic Triumph, Biomagnetic Handbook: A Guide to Medical Magnets, The Energy Medicine of Tomorrow and several other books, summarises the benefits of magnetism as follows:

- Encourages restorative sleep
- Reduces or alleviates pain
- Dissolves calcium deposits around arthritic joints
- Assists body cells in fighting infections
- Reduces resting heart rate
- Increases oxygenation to body cells
- Alleviates the symptoms of Magnetic Field Deficiency Syndrome.

Magnetic Field Deficiency Syndrome was identified in Japan in the late 1950's. It is characterised by symptoms like lack of energy, insomnia, generalised aches and pains, upper back and neck stiffness, frequent headaches, dizziness, constipation, etc. These symptoms closely correlate with Chronic Fatigue Syndrome.

As usual, the Japanese were in the forefront of research. It resulted in the approval by the Japanese Minister of Health & Welfare in 1961 for the manufacture and sale of magnetic therapeutic devices.

The manufacture and sale of magnetic therapeutic devices is now the 20th largest industry in Japan. Thirty million Japanese use a therapeutic device according to Nikken Corporation. They have found it useful for deep muscle pain, stiffness, arthritic symptoms and other related problems. Magnets also dramatically increase the healing time in non-union fractures.

The magnetic field produced by permanent magnets is a safe, natural energy source. There are no harmful exposure levels and no limitations by governmental agencies. Galen, noted Greek physician, author and educator, referred to magnetism as an excellent purgative (laxative).

Electromagnetic Fields

Natural permanent magnetic fields are not to be confused with the alternating electromagnetic fields associated with high-tension electrical power lines. The human being is bombarded everyday with smaller amounts of electromagnetic charge emanating from electrical conveniences with which we surround ourselves. A restored negative, permanent magnetic field can help counteract these effects.

Many scientists insist that alternating electromagnetic fields are harmful. These fields are positive and negative and have an alternating current frequency of 60 cycles per second. This is 7.66 times too fast for the average body organ resonance frequency of 7.83 and can cause cell fatigue in time.

According to Dr Kyoichi Nakagawa, MD, director of the Isuzu Hospital in Tokyo, the human body is under the influence of the earth's magnetic field and is in some sort of a balanced relationship with it.

Writing in the Japan Medical Journal, December 4, 1976, he points out that today, thanks to our modern lifestyle, the effect of the earth's magnetic field has decreased. Consequently, it can be assumed that this lack of magnetism has adversely affected the human body. Therefore, there is need to supplement this deficiency with the external application of magnetic forces. He feels that there is a direct relationship between the decrease in the earth's magnetic field acting on the human body and the improvement of abnormal conditions of the human body by the application of magnetic fields.

"This is my reason for advocating the presence of the magnetic field deficiency syndrome in living bodies," he says. "It is not clear if a similar syndrome occurs in living bodies other than human beings. However, from the clinical point of view, I believe that the syndrome does exist in human bodies."

The clinical image of the symptoms resemble the chronic fatigue syndrome mentioned earlier: stiffness of the shoulders, back and scruff of the neck, uncertain lumbago, chest pains for no specific reason, habitual headache and heaviness of the head, dizziness and insomnia for uncertain reasons, habitual constipation, general lassitude, etc.

"Generally speaking, the specific cause of the illness is not noticeable or no specific relationship between the original illness and the derivative symptoms can be found," says Dr Nakagawa. "The symptoms neither improve nor get worse, no clue being gained from clinical examination. Among those above-mentioned, there are, of course, some symptoms, which accompany such illnesses as hypertension, diabetes, disease of the digestive organs, bone and nerve diseases, etc. However, as with the syndrome, such symptoms continue even after the original disease has been treated or cured. So any relationship between such symptoms and the original disease can be excluded.

"In other words, it is a syndrome in which no objective pathological findings can be noticed from routine physical and clinical examinations, but in which the subjective symptoms persist and are hard to improve, resisting various treatments but responding to the application of a magnetic field. An unbalanced autonomic nervous system or part of such might be included in this syndrome."

Dr Nakagawa props his argument by citing magneto-therapy research conducted in Japan. In tests conducted to relieve stiffness of the shoulders, a reasonably high rate of success was achieved by having participants wear ferrite permanent magnet bands in the form of bracelets. The details of the tests were reported to the first symposium on 'Magnetism and Living Bodies' held in 1959. The same year, at the second symposium, it was revealed that similar magnetic bracelets had proved effective in treating stiffness of the shoulders. It was also reported that by using two types of magnetic bracelets having surface flux densities of 470 gauss, the improvement of subjective symptoms was visible without any change in blood serum fat and blood serum protein.

Comparisons were also made with non-magnetised bracelets. One group of 1,163 was given magnetic bracelets and another group of 644, non-magnetised bracelets to check if the magnets really made a difference to stiff shoulders. The magnetic bracelets clearly made a difference.

Foam rubber mattresses containing ferrite permanent magnets were also tested on hospitalised patients. An improvement of subjective symptoms was noticed.

In 1974, questionnaires were distributed with patch-on-the-skin type magneto-therapeutic devices used to treat subjective symptoms. By dividing the 11,648 cases into four groups and investigating each one, an over 90% effective rate was determined.

Using a blind test, a considerable difference was noticed between magnetised and non-magnetised rings. In the treatment of stiff shoulders, magnetised rings showed an 80.2% effective rate, while non-magnetised rings showed a 6.3% effective rate.

A high rate of effectiveness in treating stiffness of the shoulders by using a magnetic necklace with a surface flux density of 700-900 gauss was also reported. At the same time, no ill effects on the human body were noticed in clinical tests.

The Japanese continued their research with characteristic fervour. In 1976, the therapeutic effects of the magnetic necklace having a surface flux density of 1,300 gauss with another of 200 gauss was conducted through a blind test. Statistically, the former proved significantly more effective than the latter. Both showed no side effects after various clinical examinations.

The rest of the world, not to be outdone by the Japanese, has its own tomes of research on magneto-therapy.

Magneto-therapy has a long history, all comprehensively documented in the Bibliography of the Biological Effects of Magnetic Fields. Magnetic treatment was documented as early as 1843.

In 1878, K.M. Hansen reported that patients suffering from subjective symptoms of sciatica, lumbago, joint pains etc. found relief when the constant magnetic field from an electromagnet was applied. The report further stated that magnetism was also effective in treating acute inflammatory illnesses and chronic gingivitis. It does not give the strength of the field used, but we can safely assume that it was quite strong. With this therapy, the South Pole was applied to the body for periods of 10-40 minutes, this being repeated several times.

In 1972, I.L. Degen experimented with the application of a constant magnetic field of 450-530 gauss to the hands of patients suffering from Dupuytrene's contracture, which was incurable with conventional medication. The treatments lasted for 15 to 40 minutes at a time, this being repeated several times depending on the severity of the case. The treatment was found very effective on first-degree symptoms. Considerable improvement was also noticed in several cases with second-degree symptoms.

The earth's magnetic field is a stationary magnetic field working constantly on the human body. Researchers believe that the strength of the earth's field has decreased a total of 50% during the last 500 years. If this continues, the earth's magnetic field will eventually reach zero in 2,000 years. Along with this decrease, the angles of the earth's magnetic field are also said to be changing. This could well be a serious cause of disorder in the human body.

There are other factors that could play a role in decreasing the effect of the earth's magnetic field action on the human body.

As the human race has long been living under the influence of the earth's magnetic field, any change in this field could cause disorder in the human body. If the book The Earth's Magnetic Field Controls the Weather by Kawai is a signpost to go by, it goes without saying that the human body will be influenced by this change in the weather. The logic is simple: Change in the earth's magnetic field leads to a change in the weather, which leads to an influence on the human body and consequent disorder of some kind.

Every human body is different. A person could be suffering from a magnetic field deficiency even if there was no decrease in the strength of the earth's field. However, those suffering from magnetic field deficiency syndrome show improvement when a magnetic field is applied, and it is believed that at least with these people, there is a magnetic field deficiency.

The following definite steps are needed to confirm the magnetic field deficiency syndrome:

- For the human body to be kept in a test room shielded from all magnetic fields, but maintaining the same living conditions as people outside;
- Research to be done to determine if the test subject shows any symptoms;
- If such symptoms do occur, apply an external magnetic field to the body to see if there is any improvement or not.

If the results of these studies are affirmative, then the magnetic field deficiency syndrome can be established.

Magnetic Fields and Living Bodies

Research on magnetic fields and the living body has become very active in recent years and a lot of literature has been published on the subject. One of these, using animals, confirmed the theory that electric current is generated by electromagnetic induction when a magnetic field is applied to the bloodstream. Then, by placing the human chest between the poles of an electromagnet or by generating a pulse between two poles by using electrodes fixed to the skin, electromotive force was determined by the blood flow across the magnetic field. This was termed Magnetoheography. It was the first time the electric change occurring when a magnetic field was applied to the human body was confirmed.

Many similar studies were conducted in 1964, 1966 and 1969 with squirrel monkeys. Those studies, using a 100-kilogauss field from a super-conductive electromagnet, showed an electromotive force similar to previous experiments on the human body.

From these experimental results, it is now clear that in the case of both human beings and animals, electromotive force is generated by the external application of a magnetic field to the body.

A magnetic field, although weak, is formed around the human body by the active current within the body. This field changes as the active current changes. The purpose of magnetocardiography and magnetoencephalography is to record the change of this field from outside the body and to utilise these findings for diagnosis. This recording is very difficult to make as an instrument capable of measuring very low gauss is necessary for external recording. On the other hand, the earth's magnetic field has a magnetic flux density much stronger than that emanating from the human body. Therefore, even a small change in the earth's field will affect the human body. This may even affect the active current within the human body, and we can imagine that this could be the cause of disorder or change in the body.

As the earth's magnetic field is to some extent always working on the body, and as the body fluid is always in motion even when the body is at rest, electromotive force is constantly being generated by electromagnetic induction. Also, when a man is in motion, he moves across the magnetic field and, like a conductive material moving across a magnetic field, it is also possible to generate electromotive force. For these reasons, the electromotive force generated when a man moves East-West and North-South will be different, the speed of motion also causing a difference.

Scientists worldwide believe that the effectiveness of a magnetic field applied to the human body depends on:

- Strength of the field
- Uniformity of the field
- Direction
- Range of the field
- Operational time
- Position on the body to which the field is applied.

When the point of application of the magnetic field and the point where the effect is felt do not coincide, for example when magnetic bracelets and rings to cure shoulder stiffness are used, it is referred to as the Remote Effect of the magnetic field. However, when patch-on-the-skin type devices are directly applied to the area in which the symptoms are felt, the effect is referred to as the Local

Effect of the magnetic field. Magnetic fields can function in both ways.

Magnetic fields can be roughly divided into two types – the Stationary and the Varying Field. The latter is further divided into Alternating, Pulsating, Rotating and Travelling fields.

In Japan, magneto-therapeutic devices are registered under the Drug Regulations Act of 1961. It is now legal to manufacture and sell magneto-therapeutic devices as they have been officially approved. As a result, devices like the magnetic wristband, magnetic ring, magnetic stomach belt, magnetic mattress, magnetic necklace, magnetic arch plate, magnetic patch-on-the-skin device, among others, are not only marketed in Japan but also all over the world.

Generally, as a thumb rule, magneto-therapeutic devices should have the following features:

- They can be easily used
- They can be used for long hours continuously
- The user can adjust the hours of usage to the subjective symptoms
- No serious side effects occur.

With the new magnetic materials, the desired magnetic flux density can be achieved with a small size and the user can also wear them as an item of jewellery.

However, for effective treatment, a magnetic field with a flux density of over 500 gauss must be applied.

Magnetic Field Surplus Syndrome

Despite enormous research, it is not confirmed if a magnetic field surplus syndrome exists or not. Some users of magneto-therapy have experienced a rush of blood to the head as well as other symptoms. This could well be such a syndrome.

Regarding human bodies exposed to strong magnetic fields, researchers tested a 20,000 gauss field and from the results of this they conclude that, with the exception of some cases of toothache, no subjective symptoms were noticed when human beings were exposed to the field for a short time. It was also found that people working within strong magnetic fields are in good health.

The human race has been influenced by at least two physical phenomena – gravity and the earth's magnetic field. The relationship between gravity and the human body and, in relation to recent space travel, the influence of a no-gravity condition on the human body have been the focus of sustained research. But, strangely, very little research has been done on the influence of the earth's magnetic field on the human body.

In the field of biology and field science, there has been some research done on the influence on test animals shielded from magnetic fields. Some research has also been conducted on the effects on the human body of being exposed to a very weak magnetic field. However, the relationship between the earth's magnetic field and the living body is still unclear.

Magneto-Therapy in India

While the bulk of experimentation with magnets has been in Japan and in the West, there are many Indians too who are using magnets with good results. Dr Gala, Dr Neville Bengali, Dr Bhattacharya, Dr Bansal and a few others have done a lot of work in this area. A new entrant is the young Karrthik Ramjee in Chennai. Along with his mother, the Reiki grandmaster Shobha Ramjee, they run a popular Vaastu Shastra and Feng Shui outlet.

"I was a patient myself," explains Karrthik. "I had bronchial cough and wheezing. I checked out a few books on magnets and started treating myself. I did find a little relief. But it was my mother, who also believes in energy levels, who suggested that I learn all about it as I could then be of some use to mankind."

At around the same time, coincidentally, Karrthik met up with a friend who manufactured acupressure and magnetic items. "His father, Dr Gangadar Choudary, also works with alternative medical systems," adds Karrthik. "He is my guru. I have learnt all that I know from him."

A lot of people in Chennai and neighbouring states visit Karrthik for advice and consultation. He treats every person who needs help. "This is service," he says. "I do not focus on big names. I get all sorts of people, from sweepers to the society's elite. This is not a money-making venture. I am also learning a lot while helping others. The curative powers of magnets are really quite remarkable."

According to Karrthik, magneto-therapy can solve nearly all medical problems irrespective of the age of the person or the severity of the illness.

"It depends on the patient," he says. "If the patient is bedridden, we provide the magnets and the instruction and the attendant can carry on the treatment from home. If the patient is mobile, we encourage him or her to make a personal visit. We examine the patient and recommend appropriate magnets for the treatment."

Karrthik points out that there is preventive treatment in magneto-therapy but unfortunately "many people don't use magnets for prevention". He insists that with proper exercise and a little time spent with magnets everyday, all the blood centres will be activated. "This is the preventive we recommend."

About the time taken for treatment and a cure, Karrthik points out, "Time is an illusion. The treatment depends on how severe the case is and for how many months or years this person is suffering. Normally, a person can return to

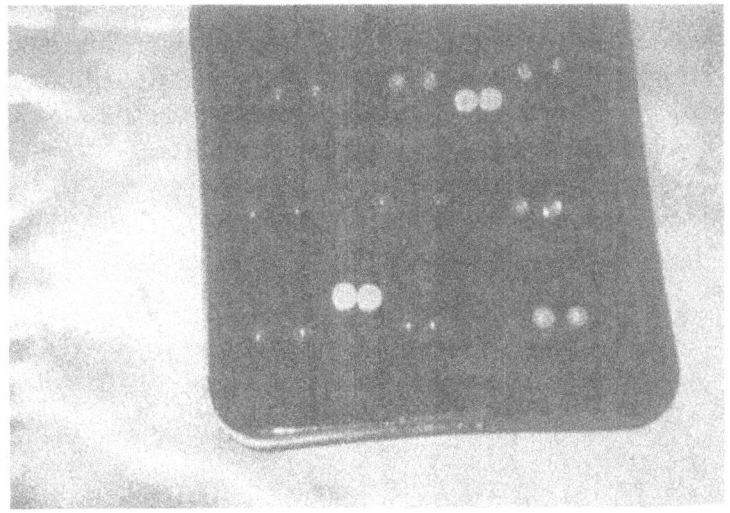

Magnetic ear tops with gemstones

good health in about a month or two depending on how well s/he receives the power. If the person receives the power well s/he need not come everyday. Thrice a week is good enough. Of course, we suggest they come everyday because that is the best."

The best part is that the magnet can now be worn as jewellery. "In fact, we cure spinal problems with a magnet mala, blood pressure with a bracelet, hearing problems with earrings and so on," says Karrthik. "The new pieces of magnetic jewellery look good too."

According to Karrthik, magnets work on the simple logic of nature. "It is based on the positive and negative fields which our body has. Known as Nadis, these nadi points are activated with magnets and crystals and this helps the blood flow where trouble is reported. For example, for a person suffering from rheumatic arthritis we recommend placing a pyramid on the leg that is paining and also on the other leg so that the contact is made when the blood flow is regulated."

In India, Karrthik feels that magneto-therapy hasn't come of age. "It is very popular abroad. Treatment with magnets can be a slow process and requires a lot of patience. There are a few books but not enough. There are a few practitioners but they are not really recognised. There is no networking or exchange of ideas and all treatments and cures are isolated. There is no sharing of methodology as yet. It is all word of mouth. There is no advertising. People know us, trust us, get better and tell others about it. That's the way it runs now."

Curing Complex Ailments with Magneto-Therapy

Another Indian, who probably deserves mention in the exclusive world of Indian magneto-therapy, is Dr Ramchand Bhulchand. He travels the globe professing to cure all diseases from asthma to heart ailments using magnets. According to him, even by-pass surgery and other complicated surgical operations can be avoided using magneto-therapy. The declogging of arteries can also be effectively done using this therapy, he says.

Dr Bhulchand says he hit upon the idea while speaking in Orlando, US, on the use of magnets for therapeutic purposes. He heard that magnets were being used to prevent clogging in oil pipes. Besides, an advertisement in the Daily Telegraph, London, spoke of a 'wizard' who used powerful ceramic ferrite magnets to break down the molecular structure of magnesium and calcium in water which causes lime scale on pipes. Subsequently, they were free of such deposits.

In Dr Bhulchand's method, the South Poles of magnets are placed on the outside of the heart. Accompanied by deep abdominal breathing, this simply declogs the arteries. According to him, a simple life free from bad habits in addition to a vegetarian diet achieves spectacular results in cleaning the arteries and helps avoid heart surgery. The entire procedure seems very simplistic but the good doctor insists he has a cure on his hands.

He adds that holding the South Pole of the magnet over the arteries from outside, for five minutes, five times for five days, along with some light breathing exercises and punching at the navel point half-a-dozen times will act as effectively as balloon angioplasty. He cautions, however, that this should not be done on pregnant women.

Dr Bhulchand normally uses ferrite ring magnets with an outside diameter of 45mm, inside diameter of 22mm with a thickness of 9mm. These would be supplied free to those who contact him directly.

Dr Bhulchand has his very own bag of tricks. He uses magnets for a number of other cures as well. By aligning a magnet with a line thread, the poles can be determined, he says. The pole that faces the north of the earth is the magnet's south. Five magnets of the above-mentioned size are used for treating asthma. They must be placed north-south-north-south-north and tied so that they do not fall apart.

In Dr Bhulchand's method, a series of these magnets (three norths and two souths touching the body) should be placed on the bronchial tube downwards from the throat. The patient should then do some breathing exercises. This kills bacteria and breaks down mucous, giving immediate relief. These patients would no longer need inhalers. The doctor advises patients to avoid sugar and milk – the main causes of mucous.

Even if the prescribed diet is not followed, the exercises will immediately relieve the patient of the problem, he insists. This should be followed by a change in diet. The food must be properly chewed. Patients are advised to drink magnetised water, which reduces constipation and keeps the stomach and the system clean. He adds that salt, sugar, milk, milk products, starch, non-vegetarian dishes and fried food should be avoided.

Dr Bhulchand feels that many ailments can be cured by applying the North Pole to the affected area and the South

Pole of another magnet to the opposite side of the affected area.

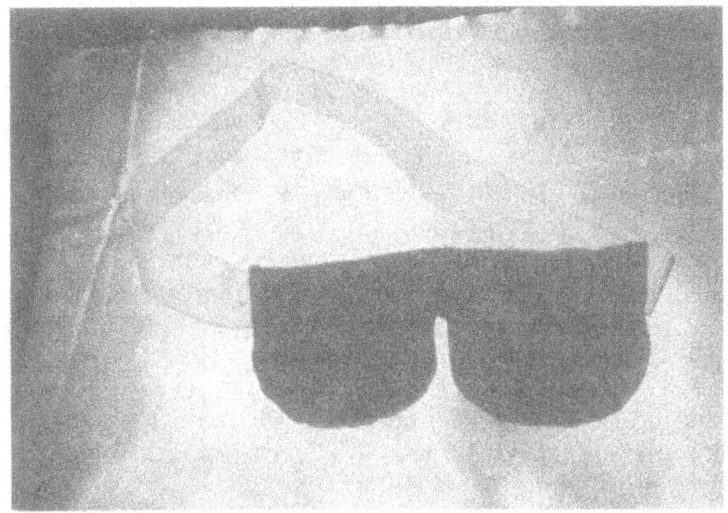

Eye belt – relieves headaches and pain in the eyes.

According to him for the treatment of headaches, keep the North Pole of one magnet on the centre of the forehead and the South Pole of another behind the head, in one straight line. Dr Bhulchand goes a step further and insists that by whispering repeatedly "breathe slower and deeper" near the ears the pain will miraculously vanish.

To cure arthritis, apply the North Pole of a magnet to the affected knee and the South Pole of another magnet to the opposite side of the affected knee. Magnets will have to be placed theoretically attracting each other and in an imaginary straight line. Magnetic field and deep breathing will automatically remove the pain. Patients should sit relaxed with their backs towards the south. Dismissing questions from sceptics, Dr Bhulchand promises "quick results".

Put some pins in a glass. Bring a magnet close to it and see how they start moving, he says. Similarly, when a magnet is brought in touch with the body, cells within get activated.

Basically, each and every cell of the human body is electrical, and every disease is created by some physical or mental blockage in the system. "By rubbing a magnet on the ailing part of the body, the cells start getting charged, clearing the blockage," he explains.

"Magnetism cannot be seen but its effects can be felt," says the Japan-born, 68-year-old doctor whose mission in life is apparently to spread the message of good health with the use of magnets. In a bid to affect cures worldwide, he also produces uplifting healing tapes which speak to your subconscious mind to keep it free from depression, insomnia and various tensions. Magnets and treatment procedures for a variety of ailments are also provided.

India has a full-fledged Permanent Magneto-Therapy Cure Centre established in 1999 at the Chittaguppi Hospital in the Lamington Road area of Hubli.

But barring a few innovative, pioneering and enthusiastic persons, who are doing their bit to spread magneto-therapy, the bulk of the research and knowledge on the subject has to be imported.

SECTION II
The Scenario in the West

1. Observations, Treatments and Discoveries

Magneto-therapy is the new tool available to patients and rehabilitation specialists in the United States, thanks to the growing demand for alternative medicine.

Clinicians in the US have found magnetic therapy a reimbursable medical expense in Germany, Israel, Japan and 45 other countries and became intrigued with its possibilities for American health care.

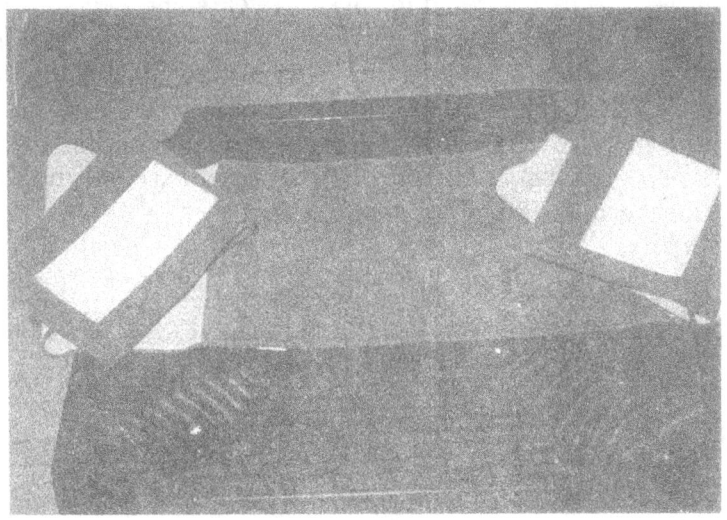

Obesity belt – helps in shedding excess weight.

Early manufacturers produced the familiar magnet with North and South Poles, but growing numbers of investigators have realised the importance of using only one pole (usually north or negative). This allows for a much stronger magnetic field to be placed against the area of pain, which research seems to indicate the need for, especially in chronic pain or overuse symptoms.

The Office of Alternative Medicine of the National Institute of Health in Washington, DC, has even awarded a million-dollar grant to Ann Gill Taylor, RN, PhD at the University of Virginia, to study the effects of magnets in chronic pain. Prestigious centres such as John Hopkins, Baylor College of Medicine and Massachusetts Institute of Technology are also studying magnetic therapy.

Ray Cralle, a practitioner in the US, first heard of magnets in 1993 in Ireland when he met Austin Darragh, MD, a world-renowned researcher, who had been using magnets to treat pain. "The joy of finding something so simple, yet so effective in helping people relieve pain still fascinates me," he says. "I have practised for over 24 years and never been as impressed by a technology so simple and effective in helping arthritis, back pain and even fibromyalgia (chronic fatigue) just to name a few. I am convinced that it will soon be commonplace to treat headaches, sports injuries and even allergies with magnets, and that managed care will find it on the top of its list of worthwhile expenses."

2. More Health-Care Attention

Who knows who would be sporting magnets now if Hideki Irabu had lived up to his $12.8-million billing! The long-sleeve shirt that the former Yankees pitcher wore concealed the newest craze among health and body-conscious Westerners: dozens of small magnets taped to his wrists, arms, chest and back at pressure points. And even though they didn't seem to work for Irabu, the idea behind the magnets is simple: They stimulate magnetic fields in the body, improving circulation, and promoting faster healing and general good health.

Magnets have been popular in Japan for two or three decades, said Hirofumi Murabayashi, a spokesman for the Japanese Consulate. "They are usually available at most ordinary drug stores without any prescription," he said. Kota Ishijima, Irabu's translator, says the ball-player has sported magnets for several years. "He changes [their position] everyday, according to where he feels stresses within his body. It is supposed to relieve microscopic muscular tension and open microscopic blood vessels for better blood flow."

Sean P. Gallagher, a physical therapist at Performing Arts Physical Therapy in Manhattan, said he often uses magnets in conjunction with acupressure points on the body to relieve soreness and swelling.

Dr Steven Abramson, Chairman of the Department of Rheumatology and Medicine at the Hospital of Joint Diseases in Manhattan, says that animal research shows that "by altering magnetic fields, you can alter blood flow or reduce the amount of inflammation by blocking the movement of inflamed cells".

Dr Alan Steiner of Denville, New Jersey, who calls himself a holistic dentist, said he doubted the medicinal benefits of magnets when he heard about them from a patient two years ago. Then he tried them. "I was told I had arthritis in the neck. I don't have it anymore!" he said.

Steiner now offers magnets to patients who suffer from migraine headaches or TMJ (temporomandibullar joint disorder), a painful jaw problem, and is a distributor for a California magnet company.

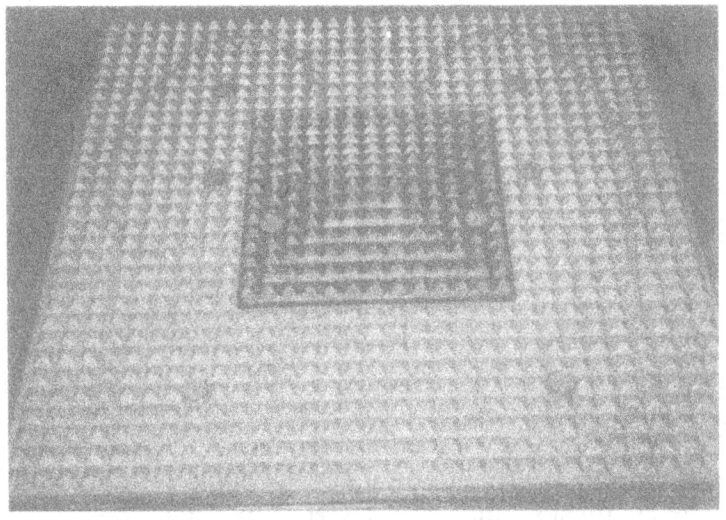

Power mat – activates all the nerve centres.

Martin Meyer, herbologist and nutritionist in the US, opines that you can obtain more energy, enhance your ability to focus and relieve chronic pain just by applying a magnetic bracelet or magnetic wrap. "Are you tired of daily painkillers for knee pain, neck pain, sciatica, arthritis, bursitis, muscle pain, shoulder pain, tennis elbow, back pain. Then why not try magnetic therapy?" he says simply.

According to him, a powerful magnet smaller than a penny, placed near the pain or injury may work wonders and relieve your pain. The magnetic field produced by permanent magnets is a safe natural energy source. There are no known harmful exposure levels and no limitations placed by governmental agencies.

Because many Americans have been fed up with the ever-burdening cost of medical care and its frequent failures, it has forced them to look for alternative therapies for their aches and pains. A host of therapies have surfaced, some old, some new. Chiropractic, massage, acupuncture, herbal, vitamins, biofeedback, homeopathy and magnetic therapy are just a few therapies offered.

Magnetic therapy has the most appeal because of its effectiveness. It is a natural therapy, non-toxic, no pills, no needles, no salves, no side effects and most important, a one-time low cost for everyone. Magnetic therapy, when coupled with professional therapy, proper nutrition and exercise, has proven to be the most effective and economical. Magnets can be used over and over, and will last for years.

In many quarters, though, it is still debated if magnets have physical benefits. "We need really good scientific inquiry, not just into clinical improvement, but long term, 20 or 30 years later," says Dr Patricia Muehsam, who studies bioelectricmagnetics at Mount Sinai Medical Centre. "The body is exquisitely sensitive, even to weak electromagnetic fields; even one weaker than a hair dryer can affect enzymes in a test tube."

3. Significance of Biomagnetism

Biomagnetism works in the human body through the circulatory system, the nervous system and the endocrine system. Magnetism is continuously penetrating every known particle, right down to the single cell. Its ability to bring about order on living systems arises from the fact that magnetism is a blueprint of life itself. All known energies have, as a base, this electromagnetic field. The latest research indicates that magnetism has a very significant beneficial biological effect on human beings.

Blood contains ferrous haemoglobin (iron) that functions as a carrier of oxygen and carbon dioxide. As blood circulates through the lungs, fully magnetised ferrous haemoglobin is able to transport more oxygen to cell tissue as well as take more carbon dioxide waste from the cell back to the lungs for removal. This means more energy and less fatigue as tissue cells and internal organs stay substantially healthier.

Magnetic bracelets and wraps recharge the body's magnetism. The body, like the earth, is a biomagnetic unit that vibrates at approximately 7.9 cycles per second direct current. Our electric devices, TV, computers, lights, appliances and the like vibrate at 60 cycles per second alternating current. Magnetic devices serve to balance the body and counter the deleterious excitement of the 60 cycles per second vibration. Magnets are also used in spacecraft to protect the astronauts from bone loss, disorientation, and other magnetic deficiencies.

4. A Small Trial Raises Hope

No one was more sceptical about using magnets for pain relief than Dr Carlos Vallbona, former chairman of the Department of Community Medicine at Baylor College of Medicine in Houston, USA. So he was pleasantly surprised when a study he did found that small, low-intensity magnets worked, at least for patients experiencing symptoms that can develop years after polio.

Dr Vallbona had long been fascinated by testimonials about magnets from his patients, and even from medical leaders. But his interest in magnet therapy became more serious in 1994 when he and a colleague, Carlton F. Hazlewood, tried them for their own knee pain. The pain was gone in minutes. "That was too good to be true," Dr Vallbona said.

Dr Vallbona knew that the power of suggestion could fool both patient and doctor. But he also wondered: Could strapping small, low-intensity magnets to the most sensitive areas of the body for several minutes relieve chronic muscular and joint pains among patients in his post-polio clinic at Baylor's Institute for Rehabilitation Research?

Valid studies could allow consumers to make informed choices. And if magnet therapy were found to be safe and effective, it could relieve pain with fewer drugs — and their unwanted side effects.

Endorsements from professional athletes are one reason Americans spend large sums on magnets to seek pain relief. But most doctors take a "buyer beware" attitude because many claims lack scientific proof or explanation of how they might work. The Food and Drug Administration has warned doctors and manufacturers about health claims for magnets.

Aware of the medical profession's scepticism about magnet therapy, Dr Vallbona sought to conduct science's most rigorous type of study. Participants would agree to allow the investigators to randomly assign them to groups getting treatment with active magnets or sham devices. But neither the patients nor the doctors treating them would know what therapy was used on which patient.

First Dr Vallbona informally tested magnets on a few patients. One was a priest with post-polio syndrome who celebrated mass with difficulty due to marked back pain that prevented him from raising his left hand. After applying a magnet for a few minutes the pain was gone. Dr Vallbona recalled, "The priest said this was a miracle."

Then a human experimentation committee allowed Dr Vallbona to test 50 volunteers with magnets that at 300 to 500 gauss were slightly stronger than refrigerator magnets. They were made in different sizes so they could fit over the anatomic area identified as setting off their pain.

It was difficult to design a system to prevent participants from learning whether they were being treated with a magnet or a sham. So Dr Vallbona asked Magnaflex Inc, a magnet manufacturer in Texas, to prepare active magnets and inactive devices that could not be told apart. The devices were labelled in code.

As a further precaution, a staff member observed the patients throughout the 45-minute period of therapy to make sure they would not try to find out — by testing with a paper clip, say — what treatment they were receiving.

After the investigators identified the source of pain and then pressed on it, the 39 women and two men in the study graded the pain on a scale of 0 (none) to 10 (worst). Then after the experimental treatment, the participants rated their pain in a standard questionnaire. The volunteers were tested only once.

The 29 who received an active magnet reported a reduction in pain to 4.4 from 9.6, compared with a smaller decline to 8.4 from 9.5 among the 21 treated with a sham magnet.

The Baylor scientists emphasised that their study applied only to pain from the post-polio condition. Nevertheless, their report in an issue of the Archives of Physical and Rehabilitation Medicine, a leading specialty journal, has shocked many doctors who have scoffed at claims for magnets' medical benefits.

Dr Vallbona's findings have led him to try to carry out a larger study in several medical centres, and they are expected to lead other investigators to conduct their own studies.

Dr Lauro S. Halstead of the National Rehabilitation Hospital in Washington, a pioneer in studying the post-polio syndrome, was among experts who said that further studies were needed to answer questions like: Will various strength magnets produce different degrees of benefit? How long does the pain relief last? Will the effect wear off after multiple applications? For what other conditions might magnets work?

At the University of Virginia, Ann Gill Taylor's team recruited 105 volunteers with fibromyalgia, a painful muscle condition of unknown cause, to test magnetic sleep pads.

Like the Baylor study, the volunteers and doctors were not told whether the subject would be sleeping on an active or sham magnet. Participants were told that if they tried to determine whether their treatment was with a magnet or a sham one, it could ruin the findings of the study.

Dr Taylor said she also planned to conduct studies of possible uses of magnets in relieving phantom limb and stump pain among amputees.

Despite a series of experiments with magnets, Dr Vallbona confessed that he still did not know why magnets worked for many post-polio patients but not for others, or why some said they felt improvement in areas of the body far distant from where the magnet was applied.

The medical benefits of magnets have been proclaimed for centuries. So why has it taken so long to do studies to begin to answer the questions? The reasons involve economic, political, professional and human factors.

Many doctors criticise the lucrative magnet industry for not investing in studies the way drug companies often do. "They don't do simple research," Dr Jarvis said. "It is hard to imagine an easier study to conduct than a magnet one for pain." Yet doctors share the responsibility to do such research and only rarely have they reported undertaking the scientifically controlled studies needed to settle major disputes about reported therapies.

5. How Does Magneto-Therapy Work?

According to an article published in the American Journal of Electromedicine in April 1995, "30 million people worldwide use magnets for the alleviation of discomfort."

The exact mechanism by which magnets relieve discomfort and pain has yet to be defined and is currently under investigation. Like aspirin, the exact process by which pain is relieved is not understood. However, no one argues that aspirins work. Now, better than aspirin, the Baylor College of Medicine in Texas did a medical study, the first double-blind study of magnets in the USA. This study established that magnets unquestionably relieved severe pain in 76% of the test subjects. The publication of the Baylor Report to the medical community has fostered the start of dozens of scientific medical studies of magnetic therapy by the health-care field.

According to Ron Lawrence, MD, a Neurologist and President of the North American Academy of Magnetic Therapy in California, "Recent studies have demonstrated quite clearly that when placed directly on the skin, a simple, handheld magnet... increases blood flow. It does so by stimulating cellular activity... This results in general healing of the magnetised area. Some scientists think magnets improve the functioning of the autonomic nervous system, which could also stimulate blood flow to the affected area... and diminish pain... It speeds healing, boosting the body's synthesis of adenosine triphosphate (ATP), the 'fuel' that fires all cellular processes... and by enhancing the blood's ability to carry oxygen. Magnetic therapy helps relieve arthritis pain and slows the deterioration of cartilage inside arthritic joints."

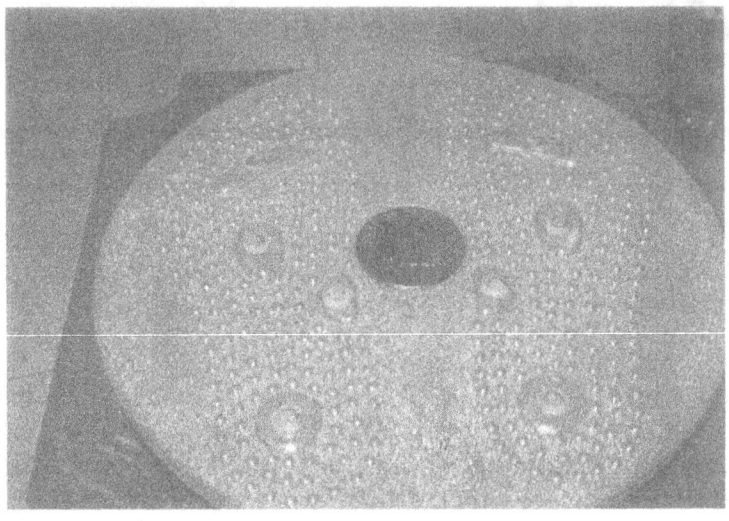

Magnetic disc/twister – helps activate the leg nerve centre and also reduces weight.

Theramagnetics, the use of therapeutic magnets, may be the answer when traditional medicine ceases to have the answer, especially for chronic pain. In addition to being low cost, this form of relief does not have harmful side effects. However, good common sense should be followed in its use. Thus, any person with a pacemaker or other electronic medical device, which could be adversely affected, is cautioned not to use magnetic devices. Additionally, women who may be pregnant are also cautioned not to use magnetic devices. Studies of any effect by the magnetic fields on a foetus have yet to be conducted.

6. Magneto-Therapy and Brain Injury

To understand the concept of energy therapy we must first recognise certain facts:

Science has discovered that man cannot exist outside of a magnetic field. Everything in nature, including man, depends on electromagnetic energy to exist. Man is nothing more than a biomagnetic energy field which lives in a magnetic atmosphere. We are like fish that live in water and have water inside their bodies. Like fish, we are living in an ocean of electro-magnetism. And we possess magnetic energy in our bodies.

Each cell or unit of our body consists of approximately 80-90 MLV of magnetic energy. Therefore, our body is a generator of electricity or energy. Conventional medicine uses electrocardiograms and electroencephalograms to diagnose medical cases. These electrograms record on paper magnetic energy of the heart and brain.

It has only been a relatively short time since scientists discovered that the brain possesses magnetic energy. In 1959, at the beginning of the Space Age, Russian scientists brought about a new chapter in magnetism. The launch of Sputnik opened a new chapter in the science of biomagnetism (magneto-therapy).

Since magnetic therapy interacts with the electrolytes in our blood, and consequently with the autonomic nervous system which controls blood circulation, many symptoms related to poor blood circulation can be effectively relieved by magnetic therapy when properly applied.

We should therefore not be surprised by the fact that many of us suffer from health complications which contemporary medical science simply cannot explain satisfactorily. For some of the more common complaints, such as stiffness in the shoulders, lumbago, lethargy and chronic fatigue, magnetic therapy can be the most effective of existing remedial treatments.

Magnetic therapy has, in fact, been administered in the areas of internal medicine, paediatrics, surgery, urology, dermatology and otolaryngology with excellent results.

Since no chemical substances are used in its application, there is no risk of harmful chemical reactions taking place as a result.

Again, the primary function of magnetic therapy is to stimulate and help sustain various bodily functions, which play key roles in the proper functioning of the human organism.

Specific factors involved in magnetic healing are:

1. Increased blood flow leading to increased oxygen-carrying capacity, both of which are basic to helping the body heal itself.
2. Changes in migration of calcium ions to heal a broken bone in half the usual time or help move calcium away from painful, arthritic joints.
3. The pH balance that is often out of balance in conjunction with illness or abnormal conditions that can be altered by magnetic fields.
4. Hormone production from the endocrine gland can be either increased or decreased by magnetic stimulation.
5. Altering of enzyme activity and other biochemical processes.

7. Magnets, Minerals and the Human Body

All living systems contain minerals in their bodies. They need to function properly. Without minerals, the living system is not able to function and will die, because minerals in the body can activate life currents or biological energy to power circulation in the blood which, along with the minerals, produce a bodily magnetic field.

When our bodily magnetic field can vibrate in synchronisation with that of the cosmos, we will be in good health. Otherwise, our health will deteriorate.

Magnetic products have many uses. For instance, in treating head injuries. Physical symptoms related to mild head injury include: numbness and weakness of limbs, organ complications, retention of water in body, stiffness, seizures, epilepsy, chronic pain in knee and back, high blood pressure, palpitations of heart, shortness of breath, thyroid disorders, diabetes, tumours, etc.

Normally MRI or CAT Scans are used for investigation and diagnosis. Unfortunately, these tools cannot find the disharmonies of energy in the brain. Therefore, there is MSI (Magnetic Source Imaging) which can make it easy to detect energy disharmony. MSI detects changes in the minute field associated with nerve activities. Japanese scientists created MSI, which plays a major role in the diagnosis and treatment of patients with functional diseases.

Some suppliers recommend applying magnetic patches directly to your aches and pains, while others recommend applying small Band-Aid-like patches to acupuncture points. Magnetic belts containing sixteen or more magnets are purported to ease back pain, and similar magnetic wraps are offered for almost any part of the body, including hands, wrists, elbows, knees, ankles, and feet (magnetic insoles are particularly popular).

For headaches you can wear magnetic headbands, magnetic earrings, or magnetic necklaces. (One company marketing magnetic necklaces provides simple instructions: the necklace should be put on as soon as the headache appears and removed as soon as it goes away. Since most headaches come and go, following these instructions precisely will clearly produce persuasive evidence of the necklace's efficacy.)

Many magnetic necklaces, bracelets, and earrings are formed from silver- and gold-rich magnetic alloys and promoted as both fashionable and therapeutic. One catalogue claims that magnetic earrings "stimulate nerve endings that are associated with head and neck pain", and magnetic bracelets "act upon the body's energy field" and "correct energy imbalances brought by electro-magnetic contamination or atmospheric changes".

Larger items include magnetic seat cushions, magnetic pillows, and magnetic mattress pads, the last claiming to produce an "energising sleep field".

One supplier offers a PCD – Prostate Comfort Device—for older men. If properly placed while you sit watching television or driving your car, you will no longer have to get out of bed several times a night to relieve yourself!

To avoid trouble with the Food and Drug Administration, most suppliers emphasise only "comfort" and usually specifically state "no medical claims are made". Some, however, are far less careful. One company in Kansas markets a book entitled Curing Cancer With Super-magnets. The authors of the book claim to have cured cancer simply by hanging a neodymium "super-magnet" around the patient's neck. The cancer discussed in the advertisement was a breast cancer, but they report that "the super-magnets influence the whole body" and "our method can cure all types of cancer".

Many magnetic therapy products have alternating arrays of North and South Poles facing the patient. One clear difference between such multipolar magnetic devices and unipolar devices (with only one pole facing the patient) is the "reach" of the magnetic field. The field from even unipolar magnets decreases very rapidly with increasing distance from the magnet, but the field from multipolar magnets decreases much more rapidly. If multipolar magnets really have any effects on the human body, they will be limited to depths of penetration of only a few millimetres.

Other suppliers offer only unipolar magnets, and some emphasise the importance of having only south-seeking poles facing the body. Contrary to common scientific usage, they call south-seeking poles North Poles. Since opposite poles attract, they argue that a pole that seeks south must be a North Pole. (Here practitioners of magnetic therapy are perhaps more logical than mainstream science, which calls the south-seeking pole a South Pole, requiring that the earth's magnetic pole in Antarctica is, by the standard scientific terminology, a North Pole.)

Dr Burl Payne, who we have quoted earlier, argues that south-seeking poles calm tissue but north-seeking poles stimulate tissue, and one should therefore never expose tumours or infections to north-seeking poles.

The broadest explanation for the efficacy of magneto-therapy was presented by Dr Nakagawa of Japan, who claims many of our modern ills result from magnetic field deficiency syndrome. The earth's magnetic field is known to have decreased about six percent since 1830. He argues that magnetic therapy simply provides some of the magnetic field that the earth has lost.

Magnetic therapy is also prominent in the treatment of thoroughbred racehorses. An injured racehorse represents potential loss of a substantial investment, providing considerable incentive to try "alternative medicine" to supplement mainstream veterinary treatment. Magnetic pads for a variety of leg problems, magnetic blankets, magnetic hoof pads, etc., all get ringing endorsements from many horse trainers – and even some veterinarians.

8. Hope for Epileptics?

Stimulating the brain with a dose of low-frequency magnetism reduces the number of seizures suffered by severe epileptics, a study has found. The new treatment, reported in The Lancet, could improve the quality of life for many sufferers who endure epileptic seizures everyday, and are not helped by conventional medicines.

Researchers at Gottingen in Germany used a coil, which was placed on the side of the head to direct the magnetic pulses to the brain.

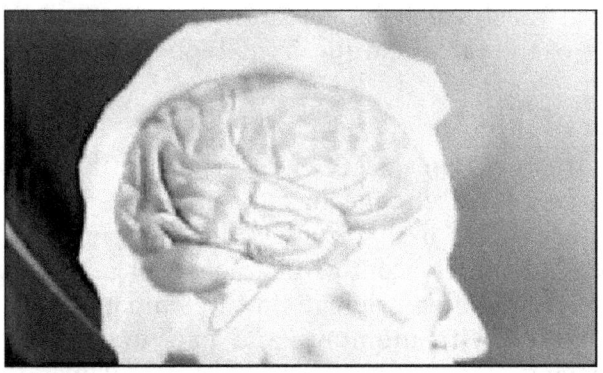

Pulses of magnetism reduced seizures in most patients.

The use of high-frequency pulses has been blamed for triggering epileptic seizures, and this is some of the first work using low-frequency magnetism.

The nine patients in the Gottingen study suffered an average of more than 10 fits a week but, after the magnetic treatment, nearly all suffered fewer seizures. One patient showed a 20% decrease, three improved by between 20% and 50%, and in three patients, the number of seizures was reduced by more than half.

Temporary Effect Only

However, the effects of the treatment wore off after six to eight weeks, and two patients suffered "petit mal" or partial seizures directly after treatment.

Professor John Duncan, Medical Director of the National Society for Epilepsy, said the treatment had potential for wider use: "It certainly sounds very interesting. Magnetic stimulation has been around for some time. The problem has always been that high-frequency magnetic stimulation may cause seizures, and I have not heard the use of low-frequency reported before in people with epilepsy."

Epilepsy is caused by overactivity in one part of the brain, which overloads the nerve "circuitry" and causes seizures. The areas most usually affected are the temporal lobes, at the side of the brain and the frontal lobe.

Types of Fit

There are two types of fit. One, the partial seizure, is associated with a change in consciousness — often the only external clue of a seizure is that the person affected will merely appear vacant or distracted for a short period. Partial seizures often originate in the temporal lobe, which is associated with memory, and patients often report experiencing a familiar smell, sound or mental image shortly before or during the seizure.

The other, more serious seizures are convulsions or "grand mals", which can strike without warning and cause unconsciousness and jerking movements.

Treatment of both sorts of seizures is usually with drugs, which can control the number and severity of seizures suffered.

The Last Resort

If drugs fail to work, other options include brain surgery, cutting out the part of the brain where the overactivity generally starts — but this is a last resort for doctors.

It is thought that up to a quarter of the 30,000 people in the UK who develop epilepsy every year are poorly controlled by medication.

Magnetic stimulation has also been used in the field of mental health where recent research has found it to alleviate some cases of depression.

It is considered a subtler alternative to the electro-convulsive therapy (ECT) currently given to many severely depressed patients.

9. Therapy of the Future

In recent years, magneto-therapy has attracted a great deal of interest and is the subject of much discussion all around the world.

In his book entitled Magnetic Deficiency Syndrome, Dr Nakagawa stressed that if these electromagnetic impulses are disrupted or lacking, it can give rise to a number of health problems: stress symptoms, mental disturbances, headaches, arthritis, rheumatism, muscle pain, osteoporosis, chronic fatigue, allergies, insomnia, inflammations, circulatory disorders, bowel disorders, digestive problems and many other degenerative problems, which cause ill health.

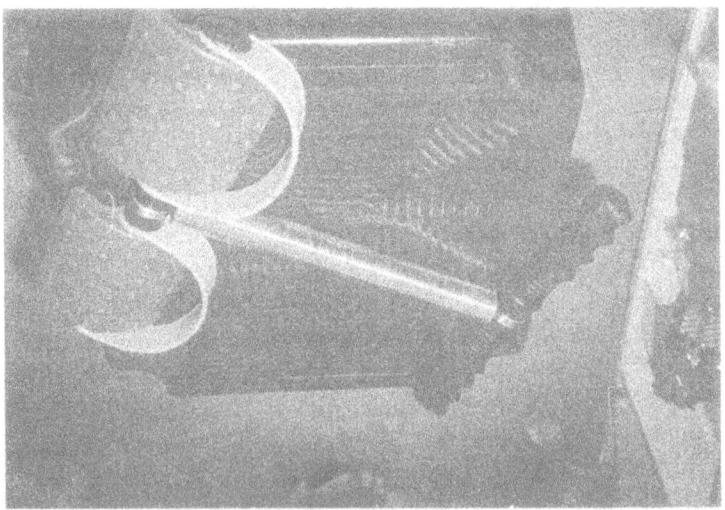

Tummy trimmer – exercises the back and the abdomen.

The treatment helps the body, in a natural way, to regain its self-healing electromagnetic balance. The entire body, each of its organs and every cell in these organs, is affected by electromagnetism. Cellular function and associated regulatory processes, as well as the function and health of body tissues, are all controlled by electromagnetic impulses. It logically follows that magnetism and its effect on the body's electromagnetic activity play a major role in health and in disease.

Although many people still regard the success of this treatment method as something miraculous, there is a very simple explanation for its effectiveness and the way in which it works. We quote a lengthy response from Dr Ken Wianko to the question whether this therapy could be called a "Universal Cure All" – that is, an "all-purpose treatment method of the future":

"In the search for such a broadly effective treatment, there is none that deserves this designation more than magneto-therapy. At any rate, as far as successful pain treatment is concerned, it has been found that seven out of ten patients who received this treatment were completely freed of their pain. This result is just as good as that obtained by traditional medicine.

"Above all, magneto-therapy produces no harmful side effects, is not addictive, does not interfere with other therapies, and is not expensive.

"Researchers have established beyond doubt that Magnetic Field Therapy re-balances altered metabolic functions, that cause pain, oedema (tissue swelling), excess acid in the tissues and lack of oxygen in the cells, by initiating tissue healing with consequent pain relief. Skin calcification, the cause of skin ageing and wrinkles, disappears. Joint mobility increases and muscles become more flexible. Digestion and elimination improve, prostates shrink and kidneys eliminate body wastes more effectively. Mental function increases, energy levels go up and sleep is better.

"Tests carried out with various organic substances in a magnetic field have shown that the lifetime of these substances is extended. Because it stimulates the body's free radical scavenger and antioxidant system, magneto-therapy is reported to be effective in counteracting degenerative processes causing heart and circulatory diseases, arthritis and auto-immune illness, as well as neuro-degenerative and allergic afflictions.

"Many illnesses can be caused by stress, but this risk factor can be greatly influenced by administering magneto-therapy prophylactically, both during the day and at night.

"When magneto-therapy is applied during the night, it has a calming and sleep-promoting effect on the brain and the entire body, because it naturally stimulates the production of the hormone melatonin. Higher melatonin levels in the body reduce stress, help to counteract the ageing process and protect against infection. Magneto-therapy is often used to promote healing.

"The human body itself is an electromagnetic machine. Each body cell has a positive and a negative field and physical and mental functions are controlled by electromagnetic impulses from the brain and central nervous system. Moreover, all life – plants and animals, including humans – exists in and responds to the magnetic field of the earth.

"For instance, earth's magnetism activates the enzyme system in fruits and vegetables that causes normal ripening.

"In just the past decade, biomedical experts have begun to realise that, since magnetic energy influences our health, it can be used to intentionally improve our health, by using the magneto-therapy device.

"Indeed, enough is already known, to outline some important facts. As electromagnetic systems, our bodies exist in balance between negative and positive magnetic forces. The Earth's crust exerts a powerful negative magnetic field at night, while during the day we experience the sun's opposite, positive magnetic forces.

"It may surprise you to learn that the magnetic field of the earth can be duplicated and enhanced with the aid of magneto-therapy devices.

"The pineal gland in the centre of the head controls hormones, enzymes and immune function, and is itself a magnetic organ containing magnetite crystals. It is actually sensitive to magnetic energy – stimulation produces its most important substance, the sleep hormone melatonin, almost entirely during the night. In turn, the human growth hormone, which is produced by the hypothalamus as we sleep, appears to be strongly influenced by melatonin.

"Without discussing the wide range of illnesses — from arthritis and arteriosclerosis to schizophrenia and sleep disorders — which can be treated with a qualified magneto-therapy device, I'd like to illustrate how magnetic energy can stimulate the pineal gland's production of melatonin and the hypothalamus production of human growth hormone.

"As we age, we produce less of these essential hormones. But high levels of melatonin are necessary for adequate sleep, and human growth hormone is a controlling factor in hair, skin and muscle mass. Its decline is responsible for many of the effects of ageing. So it may be no exaggeration to say that electromagnetic stimulation of the pineal gland could slow the ageing process. I have seen many people whose hair and skin became healthier as a result of magneto-therapy.

"Some people show signs of hair returning to its normal colour. Because of the increase of the human growth hormone, older subjects typically show an increased rate of hair and nail growth.

"There are two simple bedtime/night-time uses of magneto-therapy: You may place the therapy device under your pillow with the appropriate adjustment, so that your head is in the magnetic field, or even better, place the therapy device beside you, as close as possible to your solar plexus area. This will keep your entire body in the magnetic field.

"The idea of electromagnetic therapy may seem novel and perhaps even disarmingly simple, but I can assure you that my experiences with several thousand patients support its very real effect. Moreover, magneto-therapy carries no health risks.

"Electromagnetism and its effect on the body may be one of the most exciting scientific breakthroughs in current research..."

There's no doubt that Dr Ken Wianko's words will ring true in the years to come...

www.ingramcontent.com/pod-product-compliance
Lightning Source LLC
Chambersburg PA
CBHW070336230426
43663CB00011B/2340